FOOD CRAZY MIND

5 Simple Steps to Stop Mindless Eating and Start a Healthier, Happier Relationship with Food

Davina Chessid

Contents

Chapter 1
Introduction

The Orbital Transfer Vehicle (OTV) is one type of autonomous and independent flight vehicle that sends payloads into the scheduled track through multi-orbital transfers after being launched into the Earth orbit by the base launch vehicle. The OTV is also called the "*Space Shuttle*". First, the launch vehicle sends the payloads into near-Earth orbit together with the flight vehicle, and then sends the payloads into target orbit through multi-ignition afterburners of the flight vehicle.

The OTV possesses the characteristics of strong maneuverability and good mission adaptability, etc. Take the launching satellite as an example, the advantages of OTV are mainly in three aspects: first, it can fulfill the multi-payload launch and multi-satellite deployment, which could reduce launching expenses and increase the launching efficiency; second, inject satellites into orbit directly, which shortens the satellite injection time; and third, reduce the requirements on satellite power system, increase the payloads of satellite, and improve the satellite adaptability. At present, the OTV has been the hot spot of competing development for the space powers in the world, which has broad application future in such aspects as space transportation, on-orbit service, space debris cleaning, etc. Its functions have been expanded to the payload delivery of various types of orbits from low Earth orbit to Geosynchronous Transfer Orbit (GTO), Earth synchronous orbit, the Sun synchronous orbit, the Earth–Moon transfer orbit, and the Earth–Mars transfer orbit. It has played the leading role of space activities including orbit maneuver, vehicle returning to Earth (Fig. 1.1).

Due to the long orbit time, diverse, and complicated operating environment, the requirements of OTV on navigation and guidance systems are greatly increased. The research contents of OTV are as follows.

The original version of this chapter was revised: Replacement of figure has been incorporated. The erratum to this chapter is available at https://doi.org/10.1007/978-981-10-6334-3_10.

© Springer Nature Singapore Pte Ltd. and National Defense Industry Press, Beijing 2018   1
X. Li and C. Li, *Navigation and Guidance of Orbital Transfer Vehicle*, Navigation:
Science and Technology, https://doi.org/10.1007/978-981-10-6334-3_1

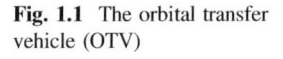

Fig. 1.1 The orbital transfer
vehicle (OTV)

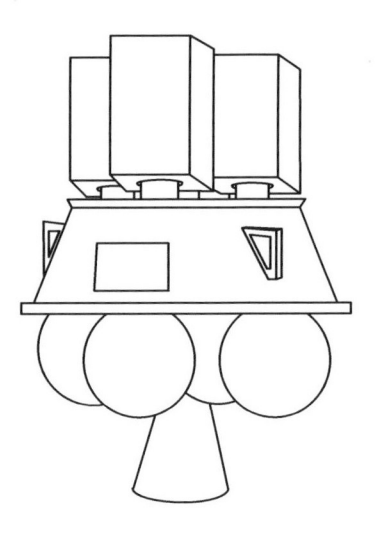

1. Navigation Technology

The navigation means involved in OTV are the inertial navigation, satellite navigation, and celestial navigation. The Inertial Navigation System (INS) is one type of autonomous navigation system, which does not receive any outer information. Its working time covers the entire flight process. Before entering into working formally, the INS shall be regulated to make the platform coordinate system described by the navigation platform that coincides with the navigation coordinate system and provides correct initial conditions for the formal working of the navigation computer, for example, giving initial velocity, initial position, etc. These works are called initial alignment.

Due to the principle of integration in navigation calculation, the navigation errors of INS caused by device error will be accumulated as time elapses, which is hard to meet the requirements of high-precision navigation of long range and long-time motion of the OTV. Satellite navigation is one type of space-based radio navigation system based on radio technology formed along with the development of space technology. Its advantages are that the navigation errors are not accumulative with time elapsing and it could work for all the time and weather, which is the effective correction and supplement means for the INS at low orbit with satellite signals.

When the OTV is at medium and high orbit, the signals of navigation satellite are weak and the satellite navigation technology is no longer available. The celestial navigation is to navigate with the celestial information measured by the celestial sensor. Such technology does not transmit and exchange information with the external world and does not rely on ground equipment, and the navigation error will not be accumulated with time elapsing. Therefore, the integration of inertial navigation and celestial navigation is the important means to guarantee accuracy and high autonomy of navigation system when the signals of satellite navigation are unavailable. The OTV is commonly outfitted with star sensor for improving the accuracy of attitude, which has no help for increasing the accuracy of orbit determination. Again, since the signals of navigation satellite are unavailable and the errors of INS integration are large, it could not determine the orbit accurately. The Keplerian orbit prediction technique could be used for determining the orbit.

2. Guidance Technology

The guidance of the OTV (also called orbital control) refers to the technique of changing motional track of flight vehicle by applying an external force to its centroid with orbit maneuver motor. The OTV entering target orbit from the initial orbit needs the thrust produced by the orbit maneuver motor, first, to send it into scheduled transfer orbit and the flight vehicle will fly freely on the transfer orbit. When it moves to the terminal stage of the transfer orbit, similarly, the thrust produced by the orbit maneuver motor sends the flight vehicle into the target orbit from the transfer orbit.

Ideally, the flight vehicle may enter target orbit after completing the orbit maneuvers designed. However, during the actual flight process, due to the affections of non-spherical gravitational force, lunisolar attraction, atmospheric drag, solar radiation pressure, and the problems existed including injection error, navigation error, and thrust deviation of motor, the actual transfer orbit of flight vehicle will inevitably deviate from the design orbit. To guarantee the accuracy of entering the target orbit finally, first of all, we should predict the orbit. Orbit prediction determines the initial value of orbit with the observation data, and further predicts the position and velocity of flight vehicle during the certain period according to the kinematics differential equations.

If the position and velocity at the track time are larger than the deviation of design value, midcourse correction technology should be used for correcting the orbit of flight vehicle by applying maneuver, which mainly includes the determination of correction times and correction opportunity.

3. Redundant Fault Tolerance of Inertial Devices and Fault Reconfiguration Technology

Since the orbit time of the OTV is long, the requirement of reliability on the INS is increasingly higher, and the redundant fault tolerance and reconfiguration methods are the effective measures for improving reliability. In case the system fails, the redundant devices and algorithm could be used for fault detection and reconfiguration, and reach the purpose of absorbing or isolating the fault. Along with the development of control theory and computer technology, improving the reliability of INS with redundant technology has been one of the research hotspots of navigation technological development trend.

The OTV could meet the demands of various launch missions, which has greatly increased the flexibility of rocket launching mission. It has been widely stressed by the space powers in the world. The US and Russia began developing OTV from the late of 1950s and 1960s successively, that is, the upper state technology. They have developed tens of advanced upper stage. Later, Europe began developing the upper stage with high performance, good adaptability, and stronger market competitiveness.

China began the research of the upper stage at the initial of 1990s. The *"Expedition One"* was the upper stage by applying liquid propellant for the first time in China. Its working time on orbit reached to 6.5 h. On March 30, 2015, in Xichang Satellite Launch Center, the *"Expedition One"* upper stage was launched by Long March C launch vehicle. Through multi-autonomous orbit maneuver, it succeeded in sending the new-generation BeiDou navigation satellite into the Earth synchronous orbit, which meant that the *"Space Shuttle"* in real sense has started its space travel, and on July 25 of the year, two BeiDou satellites were sent into orbit and realized the double payloads launching, which symbolizes that the BeiDou satellite navigation system has taken one solid step toward the goal of covering the whole globe.

Chapter 2
Modeling and Hardware Components of Control System of the OTV

2.1 Introduction

The design of navigation and guidance system of the OTV is carried out on the basis of the kinetic equations and dynamic equations of the control object. This chapter takes the OTV as the control object first, defines the coordinate system, analyzes the forces acting on the flight vehicle, and establishes the kinetics motion equation. In addition, it discusses the hardware components of control system of fight vehicle as well.

2.2 System of Coordinate Systems

2.2.1 System of Proprio-coordinate

Definition of the system of proprio-coordinate $O_bX_bY_bZ_b$: the system of proprio-coordinate is one type of dynamic coordinate system that is connected to flight vehicle and moves along with the vehicle. Its origin is at the centroid of the flight vehicle. The O_bX_b-axis is parallel to the fuselage axis and points forward within the symmetrical plane of flight vehicle. The O_bZ_b-axis is also inside the symmetrical plane and perpendicular to the O_bX_b-axis and points downward. The O_bY_b-axis is perpendicular to the symmetrical plane and points rightward.

2.2.2 Geocentric Inertial Coordinate System

Definition of geocentric inertial coordinate system $O_eX_iY_iZ_i$: the origin of such coordinate system is at the geocentric, the $O_e.O_eX_i$-axis in equatorial plane points at

© Springer Nature Singapore Pte Ltd. and National Defense Industry Press, Beijing 2018
X. Li and C. Li, *Navigation and Guidance of Orbital Transfer Vehicle*, Navigation: Science and Technology, https://doi.org/10.1007/978-981-10-6334-3_2

the mean equinox, the O_eZ_i-axis is perpendicular to the equatorial plane and coincides with the Earth rotation direction, and the O_eY_i-axis is determined according to right-handed coordinate system.

2.2.3   Launching Coordinate System

Definition of launching coordinate system $OXYZ$: the coordinate origin coincides with the launch point O, that is, the OX-axis in the horizontal plane of launching point points at the launching direction. The OY-axis points at upward, that is, perpendicular to the horizon of launching point. The OZ- axis is perpendicular to the OXY plane and forms the right-handed coordinate system. Since the launching point O rotates with the Earth, the launching coordinate system is the one moving coordinate system.

2.2.4   Launching Inertial System

Definition of launching inertial coordinate system $O_aX_aY_aZ_a$: At the instant of flight vehicle takes off, the origin O_a coincides with the launching point, and the axles are coinciding with that of the launching coordinate system. After the flight vehicle takes off, the origin O_a and the axial directions of the coordinate system are kept static in inertial space.

2.2.5   Orbital Coordinate System of Injection Point

The orbital coordinate system of injection point $O_{ocf}X_{ocf}Y_{ocf}Z_{ocf}$: the origin is selected at the geocentric, the OY_{ocf}-axis is the joint line between the geocentric and injection point upward positive (that is away from the Earth), OX_{ocf}-axis is perpendicular to OY_{ocf}-axis, and parallel to the local level of the injection point, pointing at the motional direction of the flight vehicle. The OZ_{ocf}-axis, OX_{ocf}-axis, and OY_{ocf}-axis make up the right-hand rule.

2.2.6   Relations of Coordinate System Transformation

(1) From Launching Coordinate System to Launching Inertial Coordinate System

The transformational matrix from launching coordinate system to launching inertial coordinate system is shown with A_{lcf}^{acf},

$$A_{lcf}^{acf} = D^{\mathrm{T}} \bullet M_Z^{\mathrm{T}}(\omega_0 t) \bullet D \qquad (2.2.1)$$

Here, the superscript T represents the transposition, M_Z represents the rotation along Z-axis (Similarly, M_Y and M_X represent rotation along Y-axis and X-axis respectively, ω_0 is the angular velocity of the Earth, D is the matrix related to launching azimuth A_0 and launching latitude B_0, and the specific mode refers to the documentation [14]).

(2) Transformational matrix from launching inertial coordinate system to the orbital coordinate system of injection point is shown with A_{acf}^{ocf},

$$A_{acf}^{ocf} = M_Z(-U) \bullet M_Y(i) \bullet M_Z(-\Delta\Omega) \bullet M_Y(-90°) \bullet M_Z(B_0) \bullet M_Y(A_0) \qquad (2.2.2)$$

Here, $\Delta\Omega$ is the difference between the right ascension of ascending node Ω and the right ascension in OY-axis of the launching inertial coordinate system, i is the orbit inclination, and U is the geocentric angle, that is, the argument of latitude.

(3) Transformational matrix from launching inertial coordinate system to the system of proprio-coordinate is shown with A_{acf}^{bcf}:

$$A_{acf}^{bcf} = M_X(\gamma) \bullet M_Y(\psi) \bullet M_Z(\varphi) \qquad (2.2.3)$$

Here, φ is the pitch angle, ψ is the yaw angle, and γ is the roll angle.

(4) Transformational matrix from geocentric inertial coordinate system to launching inertial coordinate system is shown with A_{ecf}^{acf},

$$A_{ecf}^{acf} = M_Y(-90° - A_0) \bullet M_X(B_0) \bullet M_Z(\lambda_0 - 90°) \bullet M_Z(\Omega_G) \qquad (2.2.4)$$

Here, Ω_G is the included angle between the $O_E X_i$- and $O_E X_E$-axes of the geocentric coordinate system, related to the moment of launching (the definition of the geocentric coordinate system refers to the documentation [14]).

2.3   Mechanical Model

In analyzing the load of the OTV, take it as the mass point. The mass-center dynamics equation is

$$m\frac{dv_a}{dt} = G + G_2 + P \qquad\qquad (2.3.1)$$

Here, m is the mass of flight vehicle, v_a is the absolute velocity vector of the mass-center of flight vehicle, the resultant external force acted are the engine thrust P, gravitational attraction G, and solar–lunar perturbation gravity G_2. When the motor does not work, the external forces acting on the flight vehicle are the gravitational attraction and solar–lunar perturbation gravity.

1. Gravitational attraction

Within the range of flight height of the OTV, the gravitational attraction is the important external force, whose volume is related to the orbital height.

2. Solar–lunar gravity

When the flight vehicle revolves around the Earth, it is affected not only by the central body—the Earth— but also by the gravity of the Moon and the Sun. Here, other celestial bodies beyond the central celestial body are called perturbed celestial body. The flight vehicle is called disturbed body. The central celestial body and disturbed body are taken as the mass point.

3. Engine thrust

The control force of the OTV is provided by the sustainer motor, which fulfills ignition action according to the control command, produces thrust to change the flight track of the OTV, realizes orbital maneuver, and tracks the brake. Before the sustainer motor is ignited, it needs to adjust the attitude of vehicle to correct the thrust direction of the motor. The task of adjusting attitude is fulfilled by attitude control nozzle.

Besides this, the flight vehicle is also loaded by the external forces including thin atmospheric drag, solar radiation pressure, tide perturbation, and the third problem gravitational perturbation, since the magnitudes of these external forces are basically between $10^{-15} \sim 10^{-12} km/s^2$, whose influence is usually omitted.

2.4 Equations of Motion

2.4.1 Mass-Center Dynamics and Kinematics Equation

Set up the mass-center dynamic equation in the launching inertial system and present the following formulas directly without derivation:

$$m \begin{bmatrix} \dfrac{\mathrm{d}v_{xicf}}{\mathrm{d}t} \\[2mm] \dfrac{\mathrm{d}v_{yicf}}{\mathrm{d}t} \\[2mm] \dfrac{\mathrm{d}v_{zicf}}{\mathrm{d}t} \end{bmatrix} = \left(A_{icf}^{bcf}\right)^{\mathrm{T}} \begin{bmatrix} F + F_{cicfx} \\ F_{cicfy} \\ F_{cicfz} \end{bmatrix} + m\frac{g_r'}{r}\begin{bmatrix} x_{icf} \\ y_{icf} \\ z_{icf} \end{bmatrix} + m\frac{g_{\omega e}}{\omega_0}\begin{bmatrix} \omega_{0xicf} \\ \omega_{0yicf} \\ \omega_{0zicf} \end{bmatrix}. \qquad (2.4.1)$$

Here, F is the engine thrust. Assuming it as constant, $\begin{bmatrix} F_{cicfx} & F_{cicfy} & F_{cicfz} \end{bmatrix}^{\mathrm{T}}$ is the thrust of attitude control engine, $m\frac{g_r'}{r}\begin{bmatrix} x_{icf} & y_{icf} & z_{icf} \end{bmatrix}^{\mathrm{T}} + m\frac{g_{\omega e}}{\omega_0}\begin{bmatrix} \omega_{0xicf} & \omega_{0yicf} & \omega_{0zicf} \end{bmatrix}^{\mathrm{T}}$ is the component of gravitational acceleration in launching inertial coordinate system when takes the Earth as the ellipsoid, and $\begin{bmatrix} F_{kx1icf}' & F_{ky1icf}' & F_{kz1icf}' \end{bmatrix}^{\mathrm{T}}$ is the additional quantity caused by the second consumption of engine.

The mass-center motional equation is

$$\begin{cases} \dfrac{\mathrm{d}x_{icf}}{\mathrm{d}t} = v_{xicf} \\[2mm] \dfrac{\mathrm{d}y_{icf}}{\mathrm{d}t} = v_{yicf} \\[2mm] \dfrac{\mathrm{d}z_{icf}}{\mathrm{d}t} = v_{zicf} \end{cases} \qquad (2.4.2)$$

Thus, all the mass-center translation dynamics and kinetics equations have been given.

2.4.2 Around Mass-Center Dynamics and Kinematics Equation

Establish the rotation around mass-center dynamics equation in body coordinate system and present the following directly without derivation:

$$\begin{bmatrix} I_{xbcf} & 0 & 0 \\ 0 & I_{ybcf} & 0 \\ 0 & 0 & I_{zbcf} \end{bmatrix} \begin{bmatrix} \dot{\omega}_{xbcf} \\ \dot{\omega}_{ybcf} \\ \dot{\omega}_{zbcf} \end{bmatrix} = -\begin{bmatrix} (I_{z1} - I_{y1})\omega_{zbcf}\omega_{ycf} \\ (I_{x1} - I_{z1})\omega_{xbcf}\omega_{zcf} \\ (I_{y1} - I_{x1})\omega_{ybcf}\omega_{xcf} \end{bmatrix} + \begin{bmatrix} M_{xcbcf} \\ M_{ycbcf} \\ M_{zcbcf} \end{bmatrix}. \qquad (2.4.3)$$

Here, the definitions of the expressions are as follows:

$\begin{bmatrix} I_{xbcf} & 0 & 0 \\ 0 & I_{ybcf} & 0 \\ 0 & 0 & I_{zbcf} \end{bmatrix}$ is the inertia matrix of the OTV in body coordinate system.

$\begin{bmatrix} \dot{\omega}_{xbcf} & \dot{\omega}_{ybcf} & \dot{\omega}_{zbcf} \end{bmatrix}^{\mathrm{T}}$ is the component of angular acceleration of the OTV in body coordinate system.

$[\omega_{xbcf} \quad \omega_{ybcf} \quad \omega_{zbcf}]^{\mathrm{T}}$ is the component of angular acceleration of the OTV in body coordinate system.

$[M_{xcbcf} \quad M_{ycbcf} \quad M_{zcbcf}]^{\mathrm{T}}$ is the control torque produced by the control actuator of the OTV.

The rotation around mass-center kinematics equation is as follows:

$$
\begin{bmatrix} \dot{\gamma} \\ \dot{\psi} \\ \dot{\theta} \end{bmatrix} = \begin{bmatrix} 1 & \sin\gamma\,\tan\psi & \cos\gamma\,\tan\psi \\ 0 & \cos\gamma & -\sin\gamma \\ 0 & \sin\gamma/cos\psi & \cos\gamma/cos\psi \end{bmatrix} \begin{bmatrix} \omega_{nbx}^{b} \\ \omega_{nby}^{b} \\ \omega_{nbz}^{b} \end{bmatrix}.
\tag{2.4.4}
$$

Here, γ, ψ, and θ are the three Eulerian angles.

2.4.3 Orbital Elements

The position and velocity of flight vehicle, besides shown with the numerical integration of mass-center kinematics equation, could also be expressed by the analytic method of orbital elements. The six orbital elements corresponding to the position and velocity vectors are the major semi-axis a, eccentricity e, inclination of orbit i, right ascension of ascending node Ω, argument of perigee ω, and eccentric anomaly E. The basic equations are

$$
\begin{cases}
\frac{da}{dt} = \frac{2}{n\sqrt{1-e^2}}[e(S\,\sin f + T\,\cos f) + T] \\
\frac{de}{dt} = \frac{\sqrt{1-e^2}}{na}[(S\,\sin f + T\,\cos f) + T\,\cos E] \\
\frac{di}{dt} = \left(\frac{rW}{na^2\sqrt{1-e^2}}\right)\cos(f+\omega) \\
\frac{d\omega}{dt} = -\cos i\frac{d\Omega}{dt} + \frac{1}{nae}\left[\sqrt{1-e^2}(-S\,\cos f + T\,\sin f) + T\,\sin E\right] \\
\frac{dE}{dt} = \frac{a}{r}\left[n - \sqrt{1-e^2}\left(\frac{d\omega}{dt} + \cos i\frac{d\Omega}{dt}\right) + \sin E\left(\frac{de}{dt}\right)\right] - \frac{2}{na}S
\end{cases}
\tag{2.4.5}
$$

Here, $n = \sqrt{\mu}a^{-3/2}$, μ is the gravitational constant, f is the true anomaly, while $\sin f$ and $\cos f$ may be given by $\sin E$ and $\cos E$, that is,

$$
\begin{cases}
r\,\sin f = a\sqrt{1-e^2}\,\sin E \\
r\,\cos f = a(\cos E - e) \\
r = a(1 - e\,\cos E)
\end{cases}
\tag{2.4.6}
$$

Here, S, T, and W are the three components of acceleration vectors. The relations with the resultant external force are

$$S = F \bullet \hat{r}, T = F \bullet \hat{t}, W = F \bullet \hat{w}. \qquad (2.4.7)$$

Here, $\hat{r}$, $\hat{t}$, and $\hat{w}$ are the respective unit vectors of radial, horizontal, and normal orbit, and there is

$$\begin{cases} \hat{r} = \cos u \hat{P}_* + \sin u \hat{Q}_* \\ \hat{t} = -\sin u \hat{P}_* + \cos u \hat{Q}_* \\ \hat{w} = \hat{r} \times \hat{t} \end{cases} \qquad (2.4.8)$$

Here, $u = f + w$; the expressions of unit vector $\hat{P}_*$ and $\hat{Q}_*$ are

$$\hat{P}_* = \begin{pmatrix} \cos \Omega \\ \sin \Omega \\ 0 \end{pmatrix}, \hat{Q}_* = \begin{pmatrix} -\sin \Omega \cos i \\ \cos \Omega \cos i \\ \sin i \end{pmatrix}. \qquad (2.4.9)$$

2.5   Hardware Components of Control System

The hardware of OTV control system commonly consists of inertial measurement unit, GNSS signal receiver, celestial sensor, space-borne computer, and attitude control motor. Its structure is shown in Fig. 2.1. The inertial measurement unit forms the state measurement system with inertial instrument (gyroscope and accelerometer) and determines the information of position, velocity, and attitude of flight vehicle during the flight autonomously. The GNSS signal receiver receives the navigation information provided by satellites. The celestial sensor observes celestial body and obtains navigation information of the flight vehicle. The space-borne computer analyzes, discriminates, and solves the measurement information in various channels; carries out analysis; calculates the navigation parameters of attitude, velocity, and position of the vehicle; and forms control command,

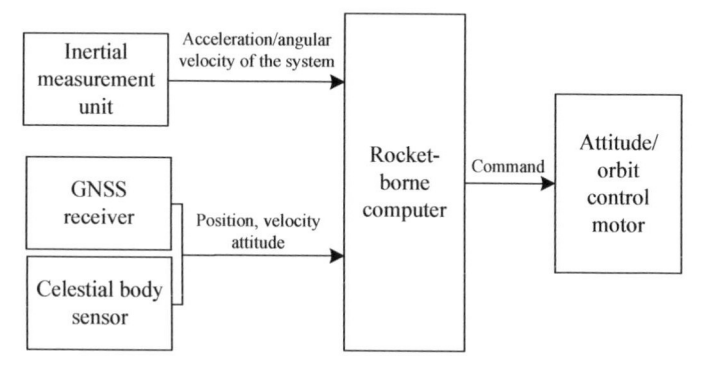

Fig. 2.1 Hardware components of the OTV

to control the attitude/orbital control motor to realize the missions of scheduled attitude adjustment and orbital motion.

Reference Documentation

1. Li Xuefeng, Wang Qing. 2014. *Design and Verification of Flight Control System of Launch Vehicle*. National Defense Industry Press.
2. Liu Haiying, Wang Huinan, Chen Zhiming. 2013. *Principle and Application of GNSS Navigation*. National Defense Industry Press.
3. Fang Jiancheng, Ning Xiaolin. 2006. *Principle and Application of Celestial Navigation*. Beihang University Press.
4. Xia Kang. 2013. Research on Hardware Fault Tolerance Technology of High Reliable Parallel Space-borne Computer. Shanghai Jiao Tong University.
5. Bing, Shan, and Miu Dong. 2004. Design and Optimization of Redundancy of Strapdown Inertial Measurement Unit. *Missiles and Space Vehicles* 3: 25–29.
6. Mingqiao, Yue, and Wang Tanquan. 2005. The Analysis and Developing Trends of Laser Gyroscope. *Winged Missiles Journal* 12: 46–48.
7. Shiqin, Zhou. 2001. Development of New Inertial Technology. *Winged Missile Journal* 6: 70–77.
8. Qin Yongyuan. 2006. *Inertial Technology*. Science Press.
9. Lu Xinzhi. 2013. Research on Deep Coupling Technique of GNSS Receiver and Inertial Navigation. University of Electronic Science and Technology.
10. Hui, Zhang. 2005. Star Sensor. *Journal of Hechi University* 4: 54–56.
11. Otiver Montenbruck, Eberhard Gill. 2012. *Methods and Application of Satellite Orbital Model*. Translated by Wang Jiasong, Zhu Kaijian, Hu Xiaogong. Beijing: National Defense Industry Press.
12. Wang Wei, Yu Zhijian. 2007. *Orbital Determination of Flight Vehicle: Model and Algorithm*. National Defense Industry Press.
13. Zhang Libin. 2010. Research on Navigation, Midcourse Correction and Attitude Control of Rocket Upper Stage. Harbin Institute of Technology.
14. Yu Yongjiang. 2009. Research on Upper Stage Guidance Method. Harbin Institute of Technology.
15. Yang Jiachi, Fan Qinhong, Zhang Yuntong, Yang Weikang, Chen Shuqing. 1999. *Orbital Dynamics and Control of Flight Vehicle: First Volume*. China Astronautic Publishing House.
16. Zhang Renwei. 1998. Attitude Dynamics and Control of Satellite Orbit. Beihang University Press.

Chapter 3
Orbit Prediction Technology

3.1 Introduction

The OTV fulfills orbital maneuver by selecting appropriate transfer points to save fuels. Usually, before the orbital maneuver, it shall carry out non-powered free sliding in large elliptic orbit for a long time. During such process, due to the longer sliding period, the error of inertial navigation will be accumulated as time elapses. Meanwhile, when the orbit arrives at a certain height, the availability of satellite navigation signals becomes poor, the flight vehicle could not obtain accurate position and velocity with the INS/GNSS-integrated navigation in real time. Therefore, orbit prediction technology is needed to determine the navigation parameters of flight vehicle.

Orbit prediction refers to under the premise of determination of initial orbit, predicting the position and velocity (or orbital elements) of the flight vehicle at a certain period in future in accordance with the motion differential equation model of flight vehicle. If the initial value and mathematic models adopted are accurate, the prediction of motion of flight vehicle could be given by making integral of the differential equation directly.

After obtaining accurate parameters and initials, at present, there are two main methods to predict the orbit, one is the analytic method. That is, first, analyze and obtain the analytical expressions of the main interference forces that affect the orbital motion. Then, predict the orbit according to the analytical expressions. The other one is the numerical method. Such method does not need the analytical expressions of orbital motion. It shall establish the detailed dynamics model that affects the orbital motion. Then recur and obtain the orbital prediction value with the specific numerical iterative algorithm. The typical representations of such method are the Adams method, Cowell method, Runge–Kutta method, etc. Refs [1–8].

© Springer Nature Singapore Pte Ltd. and National Defense Industry Press, Beijing 2018
X. Li and C. Li, *Navigation and Guidance of Orbital Transfer Vehicle*, Navigation:
Science and Technology, https://doi.org/10.1007/978-981-10-6334-3_3

3.2   Numerical Integration Algorithm

The numerical integration is to integrate the instantaneous elements of orbit or position and velocity of flight vehicle at the next moment step by step based on the orbital motion differential equation and determined initial value. If the steps and orders of integration are appropriate, commonly, we could obtain the ideal accuracy. At present, the numerical integration algorithms used for orbit prediction of flight vehicle are the Adams method, Cowell method, and Runge–Kutta series of methods. The difference of varied numerical algorithm is the method error.

3.2.1   Fundamental of Numerical Integration Method

One known ordinary differential equation and the initial value are

$$\begin{cases} \dot{y} = f(t, y) \\ y(t_0) = y_0 \end{cases} \tag{3.2.1}$$

For orbit prediction, the y in the formula above is the state quantity (position, velocity or orbital elements) Make double integral, then,

$$y(t) = y(t_0) + \int_{t_0}^{t} f(t, y) \mathrm{d}t \tag{3.2.2}$$

The continuous solutions at $t = t_0, t_1, \cdots, t_{m+1}$ are

$$y(t_{m+1}) = y(t_0) + \int_{t_0}^{t_{m+1}} f(t, y) \mathrm{d}t$$

$$= y(t_m) + \int_{t_m}^{t_{m+1}} f(t, y) \mathrm{d}t \tag{3.2.3}$$

Let

$$q_m = \int_{t_m}^{t_{m+1}} f(t, y) \mathrm{d}t \tag{3.2.4}$$

Then

$$y(t_{m+1}) = y(t_m) + q_m \tag{3.2.5}$$

Or shown as

$$y_{m+1} = y_m + q_m \tag{3.2.6}$$

That is the difference equation of such system.

Numerical solution d is to solve the initial value problem.

The numerical solution d is to seek for the approximate solution $y_1, y_2, \cdots, y_m, y_{m+1}$ (that is the numerical solution) of the initial value problem at a series of discrete points $t_0, t_1, \cdots, t_m, t_{m+1}$. The interval between two neighboring discrete points $h = t_{m+1} - t_m$ is called calculation step or step. From the known initial condition y_0 ,we could recur and calculate the numerical values Y_i at various moments step by step, thus, various numerical integration methods appeared.

3.2.2 Common Numerical Integration Methods

1. The Adams method
(1) Explicit formula

Quadrature two ends of orbital dynamics differential equation, integral from t_n to t_{n+1}, obtain the equivalent integration equation

$$x(t_{n+1}) = x(t_n) + \int_{t_n}^{t_{n+1}} f(t, x(t)) dt \tag{3.2.7}$$

Replace the integrand at right end of the above-mentioned formula with polynomial interpolation, discretize and obtain the numerical formula. Here, the Newton difference formula is used, recorded as

$$\nabla f_n = \sum_{t=0}^{m} (-1)^l \binom{m}{l} f_{n-l} \tag{3.2.8}$$

Here, ∇ is the backward difference operator, there is,

$$\begin{cases} \nabla f_n = \nabla f(x_n) = f(x_n) - f(x_n - h) \\ \nabla^2 f_n = \nabla f(x_n) - \nabla f(x_n - h) \\ = f(x_n) - 2f(x_n - h) + f(x_n - 2h) \\ \cdots \cdots \end{cases} \tag{3.2.9}$$

The backward difference polynomial of corresponding function f is

$$P(t) = \sum_{m=0}^{k-1} (-1)^m \binom{-s}{m} \nabla^m f_n \qquad (3.2.10)$$

Here, k interpolation points are used. The instrumental variable s is defined by the following formula

$$s = \frac{t - t_n}{h} \qquad (3.2.11)$$

While

$$s + 1 = \frac{t - t_n}{h} + 1 = \frac{t - t_{n-1}}{h}, \ldots, s + m - 1 = \frac{t - t_{n-m+1}}{h} \qquad (3.2.12)$$

$\binom{-s}{m}$ is the generalized binomial coefficient, which could be shown as

$$\binom{-s}{,} = (-1)^m \binom{s+m-1}{m} \qquad (3.2.13)$$

Put the interpolation polynomial $P(t)$ into the explicit formula and obtain

$$x_{n+1} = x_n + h \sum_{m=0}^{k-1} \left[\int_{t_n}^{t_{n+1}} \frac{1}{h} (-1)^m \binom{-s}{m} dt \right] \nabla^m \qquad (3.2.14)$$

The above-mentioned formula could be written as

$$x_{n+1} = x_n + h \sum_{m=0}^{k-1} \gamma_m \nabla^m f_n \qquad (3.2.15)$$

Here $\gamma_m = \int_{t_n}^{t_{n+1}} \frac{1}{h} (-1)^m \binom{-s}{m} dt = \int_0^1 \binom{s+m-1}{m} ds$

The Adams explicit formula is

$$x_{n+1} = x_n + h \sum_{t=0}^{k-1} \beta_{kl} f_{n-l}, \ k = 1, 2, \ldots \qquad (3.2.16)$$

Here

$$\beta_{kl} = (-1)^l \sum_{m=1}^{k-1} \binom{m}{l} \gamma_m = (-1)^l \left[\binom{l}{l} \gamma_l + \binom{l+1}{l} \gamma_{l+1} + \ldots + \binom{k-1}{l} \gamma_{k-1} \right]$$

(2) Implicit Formula

According to the deduction process of the explicit formula, the Adams implicit formula is obtained as follows:

$$x_{n+1} = x_n + h \sum_{l=0}^{k-1} \beta^*_{kl} f_{n+1-l}, k = 1, 2, \ldots \qquad (3.2.17)$$

Here $\beta^*_{kl} = (-1)^l \sum_{m=l}^{k-1} \binom{m}{l} \gamma^*_m, \sum_{i=0}^{m} \gamma^*_i = \gamma_m, m = 0, 1, 2, \ldots$

2. The Cowell Method

The Cowell method is used for solving the initial value problems of the following second-order equation,

$$\dot{x}_n \begin{cases} \ddot{x} = f(x, t) \\ x(t_0) = x_0, \dot{x}(t_0) = \dot{x}_0 \end{cases} \qquad (3.2.18)$$

In every calculation, we only need to give x_n directly instead of calculating $\dot{x}_n$. This is simpler than the method of solving the numerical values with Adams method after writing the second-order equation as the first-order equations.

The current multi-illegal formulas used for handing problems are different from the Adams explicit formula. The common mode is

$$\alpha_k x_{n+k} + \alpha_{k-1} x_{n+k-1} + \cdots + \alpha_0 x_n = h^2 (\beta_k f_{n+k} + \beta_{k-1} f_{n+k-1} + \cdots + \beta_0 f_n) \qquad (3.2.19)$$

(1) Explicit Formula

Quadrature the differential equation of Cowell problem and we obtain

$$\dot{x}(t) = \dot{x}(t_n) + \int_{t_n}^{t} f(t, x(t)) dt \qquad (3.2.20)$$

Make integrals the two ends of such formula again, then, integrates from t_n to t_{n+1} and from t_n to t_{n-1}, there is

$$\begin{cases} x(t_{n+1}) = x(t_n) + h\dot{x}(t_n) + \int_{t_n}^{t_{n+1}} \int_{t_n}^{t} f(t, x(t)) dt^2 \\ x(t_{n-1}) = x(t_n) + h\dot{x}(t_n) + \int_{t_n}^{t_{n-1}} \int_{t_n}^{t} f(t, x(t)) dt^2 \end{cases} \qquad (3.2.21)$$

Remove $\dot{x}(t_n)$ from the two formulas, and finally, obtain the equivalent integration process, that is

$$x(t_{n+1}) - 2x(t_n) + \dot{x}(t_{n-1}) = \int_{t_n}^{t_{n+1}} \int_{t_n}^{t} f(t, x(t))dt^2 + \int_{t_n}^{t_{n-1}} \int_{t_n}^{t} f(t, x(t))dt^2 \quad (3.2.22)$$

Replace the integrand with the interpolation polynominal, give the discrete numerical formula. From the deduction process that is similar to the Adams explicit formula and we obtain

$$x_{n+1} = 2x_n - x_{n-1} + h^2 \sum_{t=0}^{k-1} \alpha_{kl} f_{n-l}, k = 1, 2, \cdots \quad (3.2.23)$$

Here $\alpha_{kl} = (-1)^l \sum_{m=l}^{k-1} \binom{m}{l} \sigma_m = \quad (-1)^l \left[\binom{l}{l} \sigma_l + \binom{l+1}{l} \sigma_{l+1} + \cdots + \binom{k-1}{l} \sigma_{k-1} \right]$

(2) Implicit Formula

Following the method of establishing Adams implicit formula, easily give

$$x_{n+1} = 2x_n - x_{n-1} + h^2 \sum_{t=0}^{k-1} \alpha_{kl}^* f_{n+1-l}, k = 1, 2, \ldots \quad (3.2.24)$$

Here $\alpha_{kl}^* = (-1)^l \sum_{m=l}^{k-1} \binom{m}{l} \sigma_m^*$

$$\begin{cases} \sigma_0^* = 1, \\ \sigma_m^* = -\frac{2}{3} h_2 \sigma_{m-1}^* - \frac{2}{4} h_3 \sigma_{m-2}^* - \cdots - \frac{2}{m+2} h_{m+1} \sigma_0^* \\ = -\sum_{i=1}^{m} \left(\frac{2}{i+2} h_{i+1} \right) \sigma_{m-1}^*, \ m = 1, 2, \ldots \end{cases} \quad (3.2.25)$$

The implicit formula is commonly used with the explicit formula jointly, that is, the explicit formula provides one approximate value $x_{n+1}^{(0)}$, to predict (PE). Then correct (CE0 with implicit formula (CE), so as to obtain the needed x_{n+1} value.

3. The Runge–Kutta Method

Runge–Kutta method is used widely in orbit prediction for its simple iterative, large interval of convergence and wide range of applications. The most classical method is the fourth-order Runge–Kutta method.

(1) Fourth-order Runge–Kutta Method

From y_0 at the time of t_0, estimate the value at $t_0 + h$ with the first-order Taylor series expansion

$$y(t_0 + h) \approx y_0 + h\dot{y}_0 = y_0 + hf(t_0, y_0) \tag{3.2.26}$$

This method is the Eulerian method, the value at the next moment $t_0 + h$ could be reckoned from y_0 at the moment of t_0. This recursion could reckon the values at the following series of moment ($t_i = t_0 + ih(i = 1,2,...)$). The disadvantage of Eulerian method is that, to guarantee the accuracy of integration, it needs the very small integration step.

The formula of fourth-order RK integrator is as follows:

$$y_{n+1} = y_n + \frac{1}{6}(K_1 + 2K_2 + 2K_3 + K_4) \tag{3.2.27}$$

Here,

$$\begin{cases} K_1 = hf(t_n, y_n) \\ K_2 = hf(t_n + \frac{h}{2}, y_n + \frac{1}{2}K_1) \\ K_3 = hf(t_n + \frac{h}{2}, y_n + \frac{1}{2}K_2) \\ K_4 = hf(t_n + h, y_n + K_3) \end{cases}$$

(2) Continuum Method

The above-mentioned step selection method has not considered such a case the actual orbit prediction requires the orbit values of some specific points to be transmitted. This conflicts with the results obtained in compensation selection with the embedding method. If so, the steps are frequently reduced. The solutions with RK method will be very slow. The method to solve such problem is to adopt the method of large step plus interpolation. There are many interpolation methods, such as polynomial interpolation, spline interpolation, Hermite interpolation, etc. Among which, the Hermite interpolation not only has passed the known point, but also has the same rate with that on the known point.

The fifth-order Hermite interpolation formula is as follows:

$$y(t + \theta h) = d_0(\theta)y_0 + d_1(\theta)hf_0 + d_2(\theta)y_1 + d_3(\theta)hf_1 + d_4(\theta)y_2 + d_5(\theta)hf_2 \tag{3.2.28}$$

Here $0 < \theta < 1$,

$$\begin{cases} f_0 = f(t, y_0) \\ f_1 = f(t + h, y_1) \\ f_2 = f(t + 2h, y_2) \end{cases} \tag{3.2.29}$$

Various coefficients are

$$
\begin{cases}
d_0 = \frac{1}{4}(\theta - 1)^2(\theta - 2)^2(1 + 3\theta) \\
d_1 = \frac{1}{4}\theta(\theta - 1)^2(\theta - 2)^2 \\
d_2 = \theta^2(\theta - 2)^2 \\
d_3 = \theta^2(\theta - 1)^2(\theta - 2)^2 \\
d_4 = \frac{1}{4}\theta^2(\theta - 1)^2(7 - 3\theta) \\
d_5 = \frac{1}{4}\theta^2(\theta - 2)(\theta - 1)^2
\end{cases}
\tag{3.2.30}
$$

Such integration interpolation method makes the large step selected in ephemeris calculation to maintain the accuracy of orbital calculation as well, which has greatly increased the efficiency of calculation.

3.3 Analysis of Simulation Results

This section has presented the actual example of orbit prediction. The related simulation parameters selected are gravitational constant $\mu = 3986005*10^\wedge 8$, mean equatorial radius of the Earth $r_e = 6378140$m, geodetic longitude $\lambda_0 = 110.95*$ pi/180, geodetic latitude $B_0 = 19.61 * \text{pi}/180$, geodetic azimuth $A_0 = 127.8 *$ pi/180 ,and height $H_0 = 10.44$. The information of position and velocity of the OTV in launching inertial coordinate system are assumed as follows:

$$
\text{X0} = [4052.2781; -1153.2004; -103.1912; 8.2974; \\
-5.5711055; 0.3985626] \text{ (km, km/s)};
$$

Transforming it to equatorial inertial coordinate system, the initial position and velocity are obtained as follows:

$$
\text{X}_0 = [-5096.0268; 4186.3045; -526.4123; -4.66123; \\
-5.460595; -6.964057](\text{km, km/s});
$$

The perturbing terms only consider nonspherical gravity of the Earth, the Earth gravitational perturbation coefficient $J2 = 1.08163e - 3$, choose the fourth-order Runge–Kutta method for numerical integration algorithm, the simulation step 0.02s, the standing in simulation is 2000s. The flight vehicle carries out non-powered autonomous sliding. The curve of simulation results is as follows is shown in Figs. 3.1, 3.2, 3.3, 3.4, 3.5, and 3.6.

Since the working time on orbit of OTV is long (3.5–4 h),the accuracy of initial value of orbital parameters greatly affects the accuracy of orbit prediction. To illustrate the importance of initial values, we have taken 10% deviation of initial values based on the above-mentioned simulation for consideration. The results of comparison simulation obtained are as follows as shown in Figs. 3.7. 3.8, 3.9, 3.10, 3.11, and 3.12.

Fig. 3.1 *X*-direction position curve

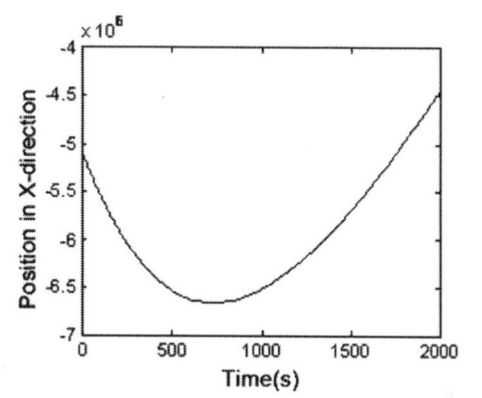

Fig. 3.2 *Y*-direction position curve

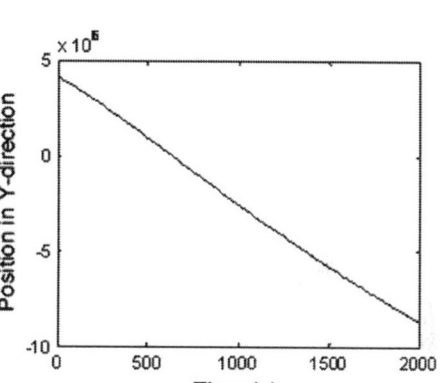

Fig. 3.3 *Z*-direction position curve

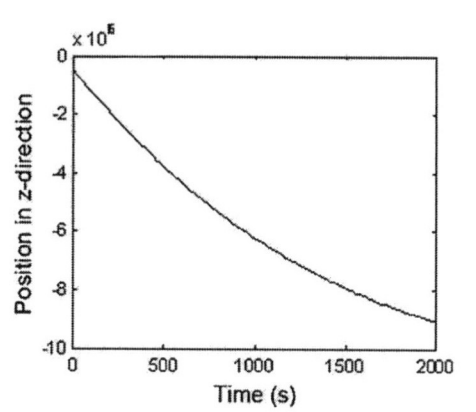

Fig. 3.4 *X*-direction velocity
curve

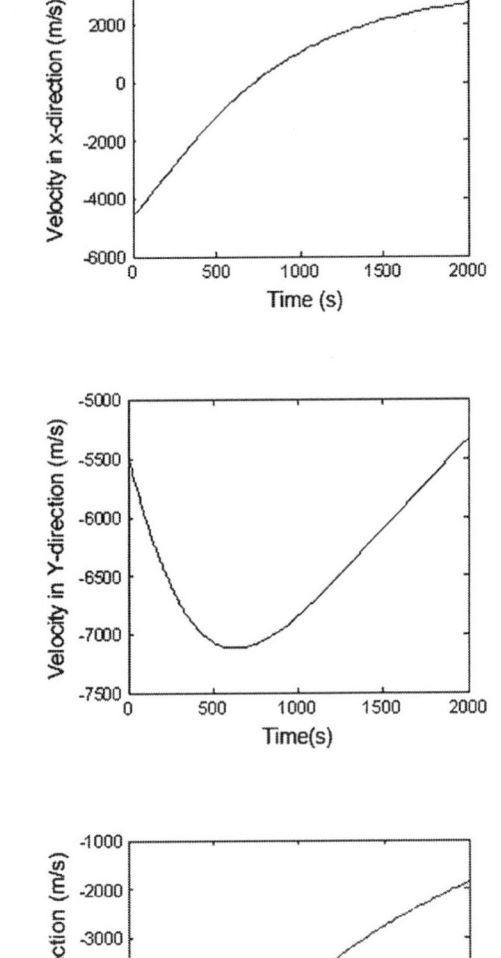

Fig. 3.5 *Y*-direction velocity
curve

Fig. 3.6 *Z*-direction velocity
curve

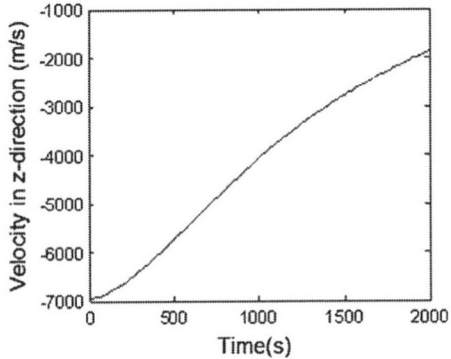

From the simulation results we can see that, the accuracy of initial values greatly affects the orbit prediction, in particular, on Z-direction position. The statistics of the maximum values of simulation contrast bias refer to following chart (Table 3.1).

Fig. 3.7 Curve of *X*-direction position contrast

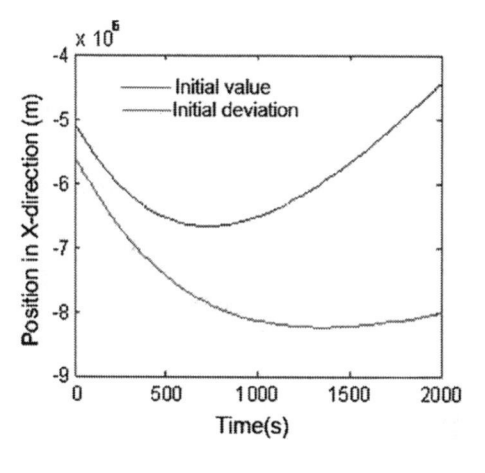

Fig. 3.8 Curve of *Y*-direction position contrast

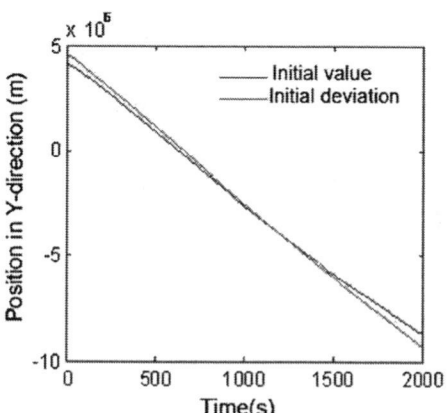

Fig. 3.9 Curve of *Z*-direction Position Contrast

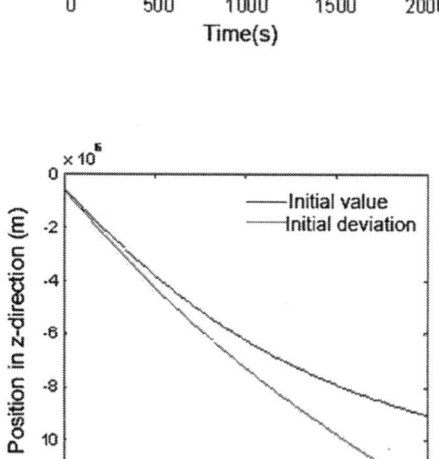

Fig. 3.10 *X*-direction
velocity contrast

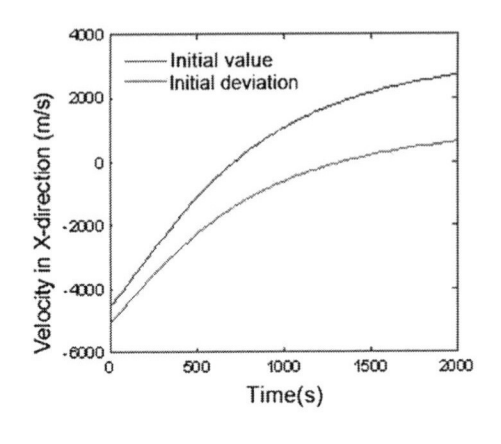

Fig. 3.11 Curve of *Y*-
direction velocity contrast

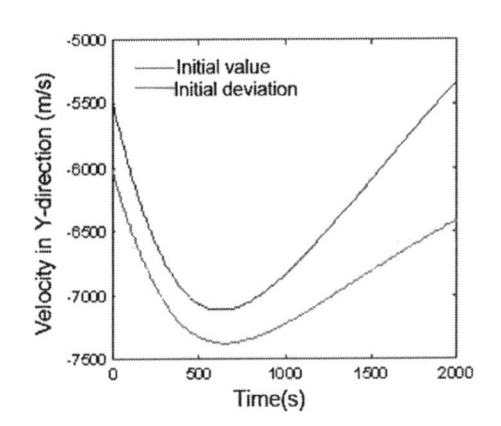

Fig. 3.12 Curve of *Z*-
direction velocity contrast

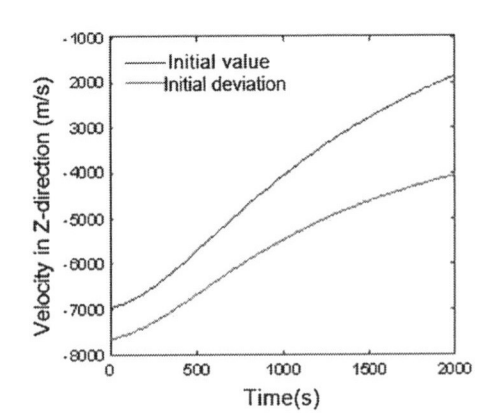

Table 3.1 The maximum values of simulation deviation

	X (km)	Y (km)	Z (km)	V_x (km/s)	V_y (km/s)	V_z (km/s)
Initial values	−5096.027	4186.305	−526.412	−4.661	−5.461	−6.964
10% initial deviation	−5605.630	4604.935	−579.054	−5.127	−6.007	−7.660
Maximum deviation	356.566	631.252	2856.434	2.095	1.085	2.177
Maximum deviation percentage in initial values	69.97%	15.08%	542.62%	44.94%	19.87%	31.26%

The mode to determine the initial orbit value shall be analyzed case by case according to specific missions. If the flight vehicle could receive GSP signal in starting orbit prediction, the output of INS/GNSS-integrated navigation could be used for the initial value of orbit prediction. If the orbit height is too high to receive the satellite signals, the output of inertial navigation may be used for the initial value of orbit prediction. If the accumulated error of inertial navigation at this moment is large, if necessary, the initial value could be determined by increasing the earth sensors or the mode of command uplink.

For the OTV, before starting the long period non-powered free sliding in elliptical orbit, the availability of satellite signals has been poor, and the accumulated error of inertial navigation is limited. Therefore, commonly, the output of inertial navigation is used for the initial value of orbit prediction. The initial alignment of inertial navigation provides correct initial attitude before the navigation computer starts working formally. Thus, the accuracy of initial alignment of inertial navigation decides the accuracy of the initial values of subsequent orbit prediction, which shall be stressed in design of control system.

Reference Documentation

1. Dong, Zezheng. 2010. Research on Mixed Model Orbit Prediction Method Based on Neural Networks. Nanjing University of Aeronautics and Astronautics.
2. Jingshi, Tang, and Liu Lin. 2014. Preliminary Investigation on Long Term Orbit Prediction of Low Orbit Spacecraft. *Journal of Flight Control* 33 (1): 59–64.
3. Liu, Bing. 2006. Research on Orbit Prediction of Lunar Spacecraft. National University of Defense Technology.
4. Liu, Yifan. 2009. Research on Low-orbit Spacecraft Orbit Prediction Method Based on SGP4 Model. Harbin Institute of Technology.
5. Liu, Weiping. 2011. Research on Fast Orbit Determination and Prediction Method of Navigation Satellite. The PLA Information Engineering University.

6. Shi, Li., Zhang, Shijie., and Ye Song, et al. 2010. Design of Elliptical Satellite Orbit Prediction System. *Aerospace Control* 28 (6): 43–48, 55.
7. Wang, Shi. 2002. Research on Satellite Orbital Control and Orbit Determination Algorithm. National University of Defense Technology.
8. Zhao, Liping. 2002. Research on Determination of Autonomous Orbit Determination of Near-earth Satellite and The Control System. Northwestern Polytechnical University.

Chapter 4
Inertial Navigation and Initial Alignment Technology

4.1 Introduction

Navigation is the technology to provide navigation parameters for the motional carrier to arrive at the destination accurately from the starting point. During the flight process of the OTV, the basic navigation parameters needed are the orbital and attitude parameters. Among which, the orbital parameters refer to the position and velocity of the flight vehicle in navigation coordinate system (the selected reference coordinate system, for example, geocentric inertial coordinate system, launching inertial coordinate system and launching coordinate system). Attitude parameters refer to the position relations of carrier coordinate system of flight vehicle corresponding to the navigation coordinate system, usually described by three Eulerian angles of pitch, yaw, and rolling.

Common navigation means of the OTV include inertial navigation, satellite navigation, and celestial navigation. This chapter mainly discusses the inertial navigation. The related contents of satellite navigation and celestial navigation will be introduced in Chaps. 5 and 6.

Inertial navigation takes the Newtonian Mechanics Law as the function, to determine the navigation parameters of the carrier with inertial sensor (gyroscope and accelerometer). Specifically, the INS determines the position, velocity, and attitude of the carrier finally with gyroscope sensing angular velocity of carrier, and the accelerometer sensing the linear acceleration of the carrier. Subject to various navigation platforms, the INS mainly consists of platform type and strapdown type. No matter platform type or strapdown type, their navigation calculations take the precise navigation and stability of carrier as the aim.

Although the platform-type INS has high accuracy, it has complicated structure, and large volume. In comparison, the strapdown type has the advantages including small volume, light weight, high reliability, and belonging to mathematical platform. Along with the development of navigation computer, the SINS has been widely used, which has been the main navigation system used by the OTV.

© Springer Nature Singapore Pte Ltd. and National Defense Industry Press, Beijing 2018
X. Li and C. Li, *Navigation and Guidance of Orbital Transfer Vehicle*, Navigation: Science and Technology, https://doi.org/10.1007/978-981-10-6334-3_4

Before the navigation computer starts working formally, the INS must provide the correct initial attitude, that is, the initial alignment. The main purpose of the INS initial alignment is to determine the attitude transformation relations of the carrier coordinate system corresponding to launching coordinate system. After the flight vehicle takes off, the azimuth of launching coordinate system in inertial space is kept constant, and becomes the launching inertial coordinate system, which is used for describing the navigation coordinate system after the flight vehicle takes off.

According to the modes of reference provided, commonly, the initial alignment methods is usually divided into two types, one is the nonautonomous alignment relying on external reference information, for example, apply the optical automatic collimating technology, etc. The other is the autonomous alignment realized by the information provided by own INS, i.e., gyroscope and accelerometer, without relying on the external reference information. To meet the requirements of multi-flight missions, the versatility of OTV is the chief characteristic. As one type of payload, it should adapt to the flexible combination with different types of launch vehicles, and also not rely on the launch vehicle. Therefore, it is the optimum choice for the INS of the OTV to use autonomous alignment. There are many types of autonomous alignment, at present, the common one used in engineering is the alignment technology based on inertial system. Such alignment technology refers to analyzing the relations between carrier coordinate system and navigation coordinate system in inertial space, processing the signals output by gyroscope and accelerometer with digital filter, and calculating the attitude matrix via change the direction of acceleration of gravity in inertial space. The alignment technology based on inertial system could track the change of carrier in principle, and isolate the external sloshing interference effectively, with good anti-interference functions. Its calculating value is close to the real attitude of carrier in sloshing. Therefore, it has very good effects of alignment for stationary base and mobile base, with appropriate alignment time, high alignment accuracy, and fit for engineering practice.

In alignment of inertial system, usually, there are two types of digital filters, IIR (Infinite impulse response) filter and FIR (finite impulse response) filter. The FIR digital filter does not have limit, stable and reliable, however, the longer alignment time is needed. The response speed of IIR digital filter is fast, but it has the zero limit, with poor stability. Before takes off, the OTV shall have sufficient time used for initial alignment. Therefore, in engineering practice, usually FIR digital filter is used.

This chapter mainly discusses the inertial navigation technology and the inertial system alignment technology based on FIR filtering.

4.2 Inertial Navigation Technology

4.2.1 Fundamental of Inertial Navigation

When the navigation coordinate system selected is the launching inertial coordinate system, the functional block diagram of SINS is shown in Fig. 4.1. The inertial measurement unit formed by gyroscope and accelerometer is mounted on the carrier directly, which senses the angular velocity vector ω_{nb}^b and the comparison vector f^b(mainly refers to the acceleration of flight vehicle produced by nonspherical gravitation of the Earth under the action of external interference force) of the carrier coordinate system (b-system) corresponding to navigation coordinate system (n-system) respectively.

The navigation computer obtains the attitude matrix by calculating the attitudes with the angular velocity signal of the carrier axial motion along the coordinate axle of the carrier measured by gyroscope, and from which, extract the information of Euler angle. Transform the acceleration signal measured by accelerometer with attitude matrix from carrier coordinate system to navigation coordinate system. Then, through the integral computation, we obtain the velocity and position in navigation coordinate system.

The updated algorithm of velocity and position of flight vehicle is

$$\begin{bmatrix} \dot{r}^n \\ \dot{v}^n \end{bmatrix} = \begin{bmatrix} v^n \\ C_b^n \cdot f^b + g^n \end{bmatrix} \tag{4.2.1}$$

Here, r^n and v^n are the position and velocity of flight vehicle. C_b^n is the attitude matrix, the specific composition is related to rotating sequence of the designated Euler angle. g^n is the Earth gravitational acceleration in launching inertial coordinate system.

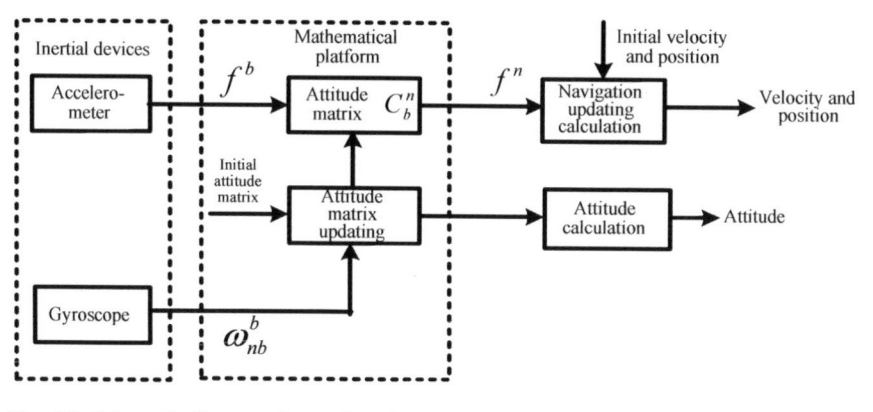

Fig. 4.1 Schematic diagram of strapdown inertial navigation system

4.2.2 Attitude Matrix Updating Algorithm

In calculating position and velocity of flight vehicle with Eq. (4.2.1), first, it should calculate the attitude matrix C_b^i in updating. The accuracy of attitude matrix updating algorithm will directly affect the navigation accuracy. Following, briefly introduce the common attitude matrix updating algorithm.

1. Euler Angle Method

The pitch angle θ, yaw angle ψ, and rolling angle γ of flight vehicle is one group of Euler angle, which describe the relations of angular position of the system of proprio-coordinate corresponding to navigation coordinate system. ω_{nb}^b shows the projection (the angular velocity vector measured by gyroscope) of motional angular velocity vector of the system of proprio-coordinate related to the navigation coordinate system. According to the rotational sequence of Euler angle, there is

$$\omega_{nb}^b = C_\gamma C_\psi \begin{bmatrix} 0 \\ 0 \\ \dot\theta \end{bmatrix} + C_\gamma \begin{bmatrix} 0 \\ \dot\psi \\ 0 \end{bmatrix} + \begin{bmatrix} \dot\gamma \\ 0 \\ 0 \end{bmatrix} = \begin{bmatrix} 1 & 0 & -\sin\psi \\ 0 & \cos\gamma & \sin\gamma\cos\psi \\ 0 & -\sin\gamma & \cos\gamma\cos\psi \end{bmatrix} \begin{bmatrix} \dot\gamma \\ \dot\psi \\ \dot\theta \end{bmatrix}$$

(4.2.2)

Then,

$$\begin{bmatrix} \dot\gamma \\ \dot\psi \\ \dot\theta \end{bmatrix} = \begin{bmatrix} 1 & \sin\gamma\tan\psi & \cos\gamma\tan\psi \\ 0 & \cos\gamma & -\sin\gamma \\ 0 & \sin\gamma/\cos\psi & \cos\gamma/\cos\psi \end{bmatrix} \begin{bmatrix} \omega_{nbx}^b \\ \omega_{nby}^b \\ \omega_{nbz}^b \end{bmatrix}$$

(4.2.3)

Equation (4.2.3) is called the Euler angle differential equation. The relation of Euler angle differential equation is simple and direct; no orthogonalization is needed in solving process. However, it has the degradation phenomenon when yaw angle ψ is close to 90°. By then, other methods are needed to overcome the above-mentioned problems. For example, double Euler angle method. After calculating the Euler angle, obtain the attitude matrix with three rotational relations.

2. Direction Cosine Algorithm

The Direction Cosine Algorithm is one method of showing attitude matrix with the direction cosine of vector. Its main idea is that the relations between two coordinate systems that rotate around one fixed point may be expressed by direction cosine matrix. The direction cosine matrix changes along with time elapses. The mathematical description of change law is the differential equation of the direction cosine matrix, which may be expressed by

$$\dot{C}_b^n = C_b^n (\omega_{nb}^{b\times})$$ (4.2.4)

Here, $(\omega_{nb}^{b\times}) = \begin{bmatrix} 0 & -\omega_{nbz}^b & \omega_{nby}^b \\ \omega_{nbz}^b & 0 & -\omega_{nbx}^b \\ -\omega_{nby}^b & \omega_{nbx}^b & 0 \end{bmatrix}$ is the skew-symmetric matrix of ω_{nb}^b.

The direction cosine algorithm has avoided the degenerated equation in Euler angle method, and could work in all attitudes. Since differential equation contains nine unknown quantities, with large amount of calculation.

3. Quaternion Method

The quaternion numbers consist of four quantities, the first parameter is in scalar form, the late three make up one vector form. The expression is

$$\tilde{q} = q_1 + q_2 i + q_3 j + q_4 k$$ (4.2.5)

The differential expression of attitude quaternion numbers is as follows:

$$\dot{\tilde{q}} = \frac{1}{2} \Omega(\omega_{nb}^b) \tilde{q}$$ (4.2.6)

Here, $\Omega(\omega_{nb}^b)$ is the skew-symmetric matrix of extended angular velocity of rotational angular velocity from the system of proprio-coordinate to geocentric inertial coordinate system, with the following form:

$$\Omega(\omega_{nb}^b) = \begin{bmatrix} 0 & -\omega_{nbx}^b & -\omega_{nby}^b & -\omega_{nbz}^b \\ \omega_{nbx}^b & 0 & \omega_{nbz}^b & -\omega_{nby}^b \\ \omega_{nby}^b & -\omega_{nbz}^b & 0 & \omega_{nbx}^b \\ \omega_{nbz}^b & \omega_{nby}^b & -\omega_{nbx}^b & 0 \end{bmatrix}$$ (4.2.7)

The quaternion numbers mainly obtain the attitude parameter quaternions by solving attitude quaternion motion differential equation. Then, show the attitude matrix with quaternion, which could avoid the degradation phenomenon of Euler angle. After completing the quaternion updating calculation, obtain the attitude matrix with the following formula:

$$C_b^n = \begin{bmatrix} q_1^2 + q_0^2 - q_3^2 - q_2^2 & 2(q_1 q_2 - q_0 q_3) & 2(q_1 q_3 + q_0 q_2) \\ 2(q_1 q_2 + q_0 q_3) & q_2^2 - q_3^2 + q_0^2 - q_1^2 & 2(q_2 q_3 - q_0 q_1) \\ 2(q_1 q_3 - q_0 q_2) & 2(q_2 q_3 + q_0 q_1) & q_3^2 - q_2^2 - q_1^2 + q_0^2 \end{bmatrix}$$

4.2.3 Analysis on Error of SINS

Because the inertial devices (gyroscope and accelerometer) have error of measurement, the velocity, position, and attitude error produced by integration will be continuously accumulated along with time elapses. Therefore, as for the long-term flight mission of the OTV, the accumulated error of INS must be corrected to ensure the navigation accuracy. Therefore, commonly, other navigation modes are introduced to assist the inertial navigation, and make up the integrated navigation system. The premise of forming integrated navigation system is to know the error characteristics of INS. Through error analysis of the INS, we could reveal the process of navigation error changing along with time elapses, and easy for the design of integrated navigation system. Following, we will mainly introduce the error characteristics of INS, the contents about integrated navigation will be discussed in Chaps. 5 and 6.

1. Attitude Error Equation

Assume $\phi = [\phi_x \ \phi_y \ \phi_z]^{\mathrm{T}}$ is the error angle between mathematical platform and actual navigation coordinate system, i.e., the attitude misalignment angle. From Eq. (4.2.4) we can know that, the attitude transformation matrix $\tilde{C}_b^n$ output by the INS actually have following relations with the ideal attitude transformation matrix C_b^n

$$\tilde{C}_b^n = C_b^n + \delta C_b^n = (I - \phi^{\times})C_b^n \tag{4.2.8}$$

Here, the $\phi^{\times}$ is the skew-symmetrical matrix ϕ. In terms of the measurement noise of gyroscope, omitted the error between linear term and quadric term, the final attitude error equation is

$$\dot{\phi} = -C_b^n(\varepsilon + W_\varepsilon) \tag{4.2.9}$$

Here, ε is the constant drift of gyroscope; W_ε is the white Gaussian noise of gyroscope model.

2. Velocity Position Error Equation

In launching inertial system, from Eq. (4.2.1) we can know,

$$\dot{r}^n = v^n \tag{4.2.10}$$

$$\dot{v}^n = g^n + C_b^n \cdot f^b \tag{4.2.11}$$

Let ∇ be the constant offset of the accelerometer, W_∇ be the white Gaussian noise of the accelerometer model, omitted the error between linear term and quadric term, then, $\delta f^b = \nabla + W_\nabla$. Let $\delta a = -\phi^{\times} C_b^n \cdot f^b + C_b^n \cdot (\delta f^b)$, the mode of component of the velocity position error equation of the OTV may be written as,

$$\begin{bmatrix} \delta \dot{V}_x \\ \delta \dot{V}_y \\ \delta \dot{V}_z \\ \delta \dot{x} \\ \delta \dot{y} \\ \delta \dot{z} \end{bmatrix} = \begin{bmatrix} 0 & 0 & 0 & f_{14} & f_{15} & f_{16} \\ 0 & 0 & 0 & f_{24} & f_{25} & f_{26} \\ 0 & 0 & 0 & f_{34} & f_{35} & f_{36} \\ 1 & 0 & 0 & 0 & 0 & 0 \\ 0 & 1 & 0 & 0 & 0 & 0 \\ 0 & 0 & 1 & 0 & 0 & 0 \end{bmatrix} \begin{bmatrix} \delta V_x \\ \delta V_y \\ \delta V_z \\ \delta x \\ \delta y \\ \delta z \end{bmatrix} + \begin{bmatrix} \delta a_x \\ \delta a_y \\ \delta a_z \\ 0 \\ 0 \\ 0 \end{bmatrix} \qquad (4.2.12)$$

Here, the coefficients $f_{14}, f_{15}, f_{16}, f_{24}, f_{25}, f_{26}, f_{34}, f_{35}$ and f_{36} are the derivatives of gravitational acceleration corresponding to position coordinate, which is related to the position of flight vehicle. x, y and z are the positions of flight vehicle in launching inertial system.

4. Inertial Device Error Equation

Take the gyroscope error and accelerometer error as the random constant, the corresponding error equation is written as,

$$\dot{\nabla}_x = 0, \ \dot{\nabla}_y = 0, \ \dot{\nabla}_z = 0, \ \dot{\varepsilon}_x = 0, \ \dot{\varepsilon}_y = 0, \ \dot{\varepsilon}_z = 0 \qquad (4.2.13)$$

4.3 Alignment Technology Based on Inertial System

The initial alignment of the INS of the OTV is completed on ground before launching. Because the interference factors including ground wind produce shaking, the interference angular velocity caused is larger than the rotational angular velocity of the Earth; it is difficult to extract the useful information of the rotational angular velocity of the Earth from the output of the gyroscope. However, the rotational angular velocity of the Earth ω_{ie} is one known steady state value, the direction of acceleration of gravity g in inertial space changes the true north of the Earth. If the measurement time is longer enough and accurate, precise initial attitude could be obtained from the information of acceleration of gravity. The alignment calculation based on inertial system is done by such basic principle.

4.3.1 Digital Filter Processing Technology of Disturbing Acceleration

With regard to the SINS of the OTV, the accelerometer has one ideal installation position. The actual accelerometer will deviate from such ideal position. When the factors, including wind interference, makes the flight vehicle swing it will result in measurement error of accelerometer and form high frequency disturbing acceleration. Thus, one ideal low-band filter shall be designed for preprocessing the output of the accelerometer and then calculate the initial alignment, so as to suppress the

$$H_d(e^{j\omega}) \xrightarrow{\text{Fourier inversion}} h_d(n) \xrightarrow{\text{Window function}} h(n) = h_d(n) * \omega(n) \xrightarrow{\text{Fourier transform}} H(e^{j\omega})$$

Fig. 4.2 Process of window design method

influence of disturbing acceleration effectively. According to the introduction, following is the description of design principle of FIR Digital Filter.

The design of FIR Digital Filter usually adopts the window design method. Its concept is to shorten one infinite impulse response sequence $h_d(n)$ with one finite window function sequence $\omega(n)$ and obtain the finite impulse response $h(n)$ of FIR filter. The steps refer to Fig. 4.2.

(1) As for ideal frequency response $H_d(e^{j\omega})$, solve the Fourier inverse transform and obtain the ideal unit pulse response $h_d(n)$.
(2) Solve the unit sample response $h(n)$ of actual filter.
(3) In terms of $h(n)$, solve the Fourier transform and obtain the frequency characteristic function $H(e^{j\omega})$ of filter.

The window function $\omega(n)$ shall be chosen according to actuality. The common ones are the Hanning window, Hamming window, etc. It may specifically refer to related documents about digital signal processing.

4.3.2 Inertial System Alignment Technology with Digital Filter

After filtering off high-frequency disturbing acceleration with digital filters, we can calculate attitude matrix. The following four coordinate systems will be used during the process of solution.

1. Definition of Coordinate System.
(1) Launch coordinate system (f-system): its definition is shown in Chap. 2.
(2) Longitude Earth coordinate system (e-system): the origin of such coordinate system is at the center of the Earth. Y-axis coincides with the Earth's rotational axis, Z-axis points at the longitude of the point of the inertial group located at the starting moment t_0 inside the equatorial plane. X-axis is determined by the right-hand rule. Such coordinate system is connected with the Earth.
(3) Longitude geocentric inertial coordinate system (e_i-system): the coordinate system formed by solidification of the e-system in inertial space at the time of t_0 is the Longitude geocentric inertial coordinate system.
(4) Carrier inertial coordinate system (b_i-system): the coordinate system formed by solidification of the carrier coordinate system (b-system) in inertial space at the time t_0 is the carrier inertial coordinate system.
2. Principle of Self-alignment Algorithm Based on Inertial System

Taking f-system as the navigation coordinate system (n-system) during the process of initial alignment, the attitude matrix C_b^n could be decomposed into the products of the following matrices:

$$C_b^n = C_e^n C_{e_i}^e(t) C_{b_i}^{e_i} C_b^{b_i}(t) \tag{4.3.1}$$

(1) $C_b^{b_i}(t)$ is the transform matrix from b-system to b_i-system. Such matrix contains the information of attitude change of the swing base. From the definition of b_i-system we can know that the b_i-system coincides with the b-system at the moment of t_0. Thus, the initial value of attitude transformation quaternion of b-system rotation corresponding to i_{b_0}-system is $q = \begin{bmatrix} 1 & 0 & 0 & 0 \end{bmatrix}$. The $C_b^{i_{b_0}}(t)$ could be obtained by calculation with the attitude matrix updating algorithm described in Sect. 4.2.2 according to the output of gyroscope.

(2) $C_{b_i}^{e_i}$ is the transformation matrix from b_i-system to e_i-system. Such matrix contains the information of direction change caused by the rotation along with the Earth of the acceleration of gravity corresponding to inertial space. When observing the acceleration of gravity in the inertial coordinate system, since the moving trace of rotation of the Earth forms one circular cone surface, the gravity vector is non-collinear in the inertial coordinate system at different moments (the time interval shall not be the integral multiple of 24 h). Solve the gravity vector at two different moments, we could obtain the $C_{b_i}^{e_i}$.

From the definition of b_i-system we can know, if the position of carrier does not change during the process of alignment, the component of gravity g in e_i-system is only determined by the alignment time, latitude and launch azimuth of the site located by the launch vehicle. Its accuracy could be obtained by following format:

$$g^{e_i} = C_e^{e_i} C_n^e g^n \tag{4.3.2}$$

Taking the comparison vector f^{b_i} and gravity vector g^{e_i} and their vector cross product at two different moments of t_l and $t_m(l<m)$, with the method of double vector attitude determination, there is

$$C_{b_i}^{e_i} = \begin{bmatrix} \left(-g_{t_l}^{e_i}\right)^{\mathrm{T}} \\ \left(-g_{t_m}^{e_i}\right)^{\mathrm{T}} \\ \left(-g_{t_l}^{e_i}\right) \times \left(-g_{t_m}^{e_i}\right)^{\mathrm{T}} \end{bmatrix}^{-1} \begin{bmatrix} \left(f_{t_l}^{b_i}\right)^{\mathrm{T}} \\ \left(f_{t_m}^{b_i}\right)^{\mathrm{T}} \\ \left(f_{t_l}^{b_i} \times f_{t_m}^{b_i}\right)^{\mathrm{T}} \end{bmatrix} \tag{4.3.3}$$

Through the above-mentioned methods and theory, we could solve the $C_{i_{b_0}}^{i_0}$. However, in actual SINS, the output of the accelerometer is usually in the form of velocity gain. To reduce the error caused by amplification of noise differential amplification, we could integrate g^{e_i} and f^{b_i} in time interval $[t_0, t]$. Assume $V^{e_i} = \int_{t_0}^t -g^{e_i} dt$, $V^{b_i} = \int_{t_0}^t f^{b_i} dt$, then,

$$C_{b_i}^{e_i} = \begin{bmatrix} (V_{t_l}^{e_i})^{\mathrm{T}} \\ (V_{t_m}^{e_i})^{\mathrm{T}} \\ (V_{t_l}^{e_i} \times V_{t_m}^{e_i})^{\mathrm{T}} \end{bmatrix}^{-1} \begin{bmatrix} (V_{t_l}^{b_i})^{\mathrm{T}} \\ (V_{t_m}^{b_i})^{\mathrm{T}} \\ (V_{t_l}^{b_i} \times V_{t_m}^{b_i})^{\mathrm{T}} \end{bmatrix} \qquad (4.3.4)$$

(3) $C_{e_i}^{e}(t)$ is the transformation matrix from e_i-system to e-system. Such matrix contains the information of rotation of the Earth. When the accuracy of time t is known, the angle rotated for e-system is $\omega_{ie}(t - t_0)$. ω_{ie} is the volume of rotational acceleration of the Earth. The $C_{e_i}^{e}(t)$ may be shown as

$$C_{e_i}^{e}(t) = \begin{bmatrix} \cos[\omega_{ie}(t - t_0)] & 0 & -\sin[\omega_{ie}(t - t_0)] \\ 0 & 1 & 0 \\ \sin[\omega_{ie}(t - t_0)] & 0 & \cos[\omega_{ie}(t - t_0)] \end{bmatrix} \qquad (4.3.5)$$

(4) C_e^n is the transformation matrix from e-system to n-system. Since n-system and e-system are connected with the Earth. The relation of coordinate transformation is fixed, which is only related to the geography and launching azimuth of the rocket launch point. Assume that the latitude of the launch point is L, the launch azimuth is A_0, then there are following coordinate transformation relations between e-system and n-system,

$$OX_e Y_e Z_e \xrightarrow[OX_{e_0}]{\quad 90^{\circ} - L} OX_{n1} Y_{n1} Z_{n1} \xrightarrow[OY_{n1}]{\quad 90^{\circ} - A_0} O_n X_n Y_n Z_n$$

$$C_e^n = \begin{bmatrix} \sin A_0 & \cos A_0 \cos L & -\cos A_0 \sin L \\ 0 & \sin L & \cos L \\ \cos A_0 & -\sin A_0 \cos L & \sin A_0 \sin L \end{bmatrix} \qquad (4.3.6)$$

4.3.3 Analysis on Limiting Accuracy of Alignment Method of Inertial System

From Sect. 4.3.2 we can know, the attitude is decomposed into four matrices for calculation. Matrix $C_{e_0}^{n}$ is the function of latitude L of the alignment place and launching azimuth A_0. $C_{i_0}^{e_0}(t)$ is the function of alignment duration $\Delta t = t - t_0$, L, A_0 and Δt could be obtained precisely. Thus, error has not been introduced in solving the matrix $C_{e_0}^{n}$ and $C_{i_0}^{e_0}(t)$. The alignment error is introduced in solving $C_b^{i_{b_0}}(t)$ and $C_{i_{b_0}}^{i_0}$.

The attitude transfer matrix from the *b-system* of the carrier system to the i_{b_0}-system of the carrier solidification system is obtained by calculating the information transmitted by gyroscope in real time. Thus, the output of gyroscope is the main factor that affects such matrix. The solution error of $C_b^{i_{b_0}}(t)$ is mainly affected by g^b. Since the coarse alignment time is usually very short, and the gyroscope drift of INS level of flight vehicle is usually very small, the solution error $C_b^{i_{b_0}}(t)$ during the process of alignment is very small, which could be omitted.

Because the $C_{i_{b_0}}^{i_0}$ matrix is obtained by the method of double vector attitude determination, it is the main source of the error of alignment accuracy of inertial system. Finally, the accuracy of alignment algorithm error based on inertial system obtained is

$$\begin{cases} \phi_x = -\frac{\nabla_N}{g}\sin A_0 + \frac{\nabla_E}{g}\cos A_0 \\ \phi_y = \frac{\nabla_E}{g}\tan L - \frac{\varepsilon_E}{\omega_{ie}\cos L} \\ \phi_z = -\frac{\nabla_N}{g}\cos A_0 - \frac{\nabla_E}{g}\sin A_0 \end{cases} \quad (4.3.7)$$

The above-mentioned alignment accuracy based on inertial system relies on the equivalent deviation of the devices finally. The subscripts E, N at the right of the equation show the east and north of the northeastern geographic coordinate system respectively. ε_E is the westward drift of gyroscope, ∇_N is the northward bias of accelerometer, and ∇_E is the bias of eastward accelerometer.

4.4 Analysis on Simulation Results

4.4.1 Analysis on Simulation of Digital Filtering

Section 4.3.1 briefly introduces the design method of FIR filter. Following is the simulation.

Assumed the original signal is $x(t) = \sin(2\pi \cdot 3t) + 5\cos(2\pi \cdot 20t)$, i.e., includes the 3 and 20 Hz signals, the sampling frequency is 50 Hz. Use the Hanning window function to design FIR low-pass filter, the normalized frequency meet, the passband boundary $\omega_p = 0.5$, stopband boundary $\omega_s = 0.66$, the stopband attenuation is not less than 30 dB, and the passband ripple is not more than 3 dB. The amplitude frequency response and phase-frequency response of filters refer to Figs. 4.3 and 4.4.

The original signal and the signals passed through FIR filter refer to Figs. 4.5 and 4.6.

From Figs. 4.5 and 4.6 we can know, the 20 Hz signal has been filtered off. After the filter, there is only 3 Hz signal, which shows the availability of filter designed.

Fig. 4.3 Amplitude frequency response of filter

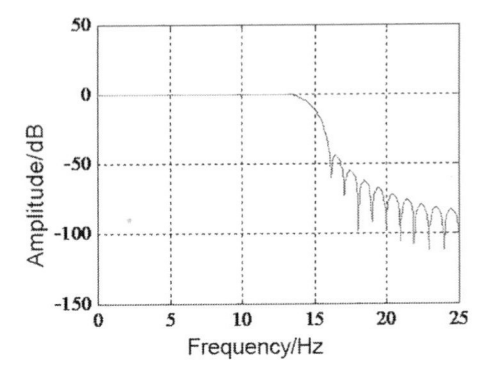

Fig. 4.4 Phase-frequency response of filter

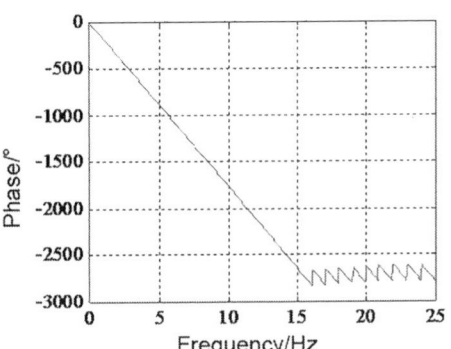

Fig. 4.5 Original signal

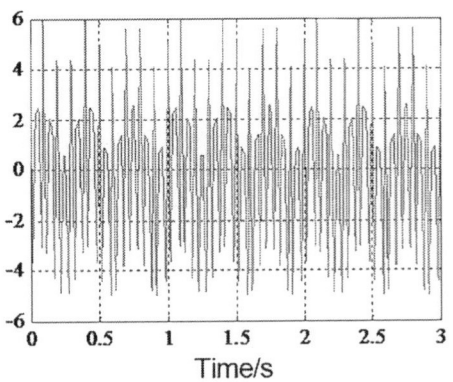

Fig. 4.6 Signal passed
through FIR filter

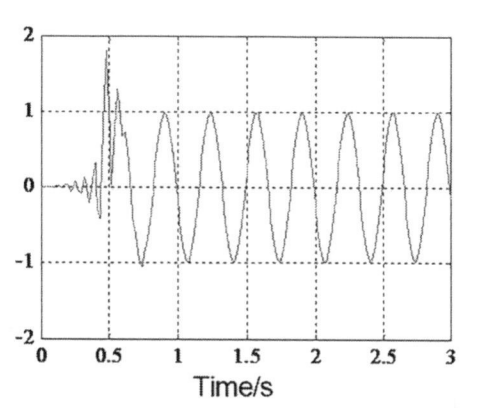

4.4.2   Analysis on Alignment Simulation of Inertial System

Assume that before launching, the flight vehicle hosted on rocket is at static state, the longitude of launching point is 121.2°, latitude is 31.2°, launching azimuth is 45°, taking launching coordinate system as the reference coordinate system. The initial roll angle of the flight vehicle is 2°, pitch angle is 91°, and yaw angle is −5°.

The constant drift of gyroscope is 0.02°/h, the standard error of random drift is 0.01°/h, the constant bias of accelerometer is $10^{-4}g$, the standard deviation of random bias is $10^{-5}g$, acceleration of gravity $g = 9.8\,\mathrm{m/s^2}$; after digital filtering on the signals transmitted by accelerometer, carry out initial alignment with the method

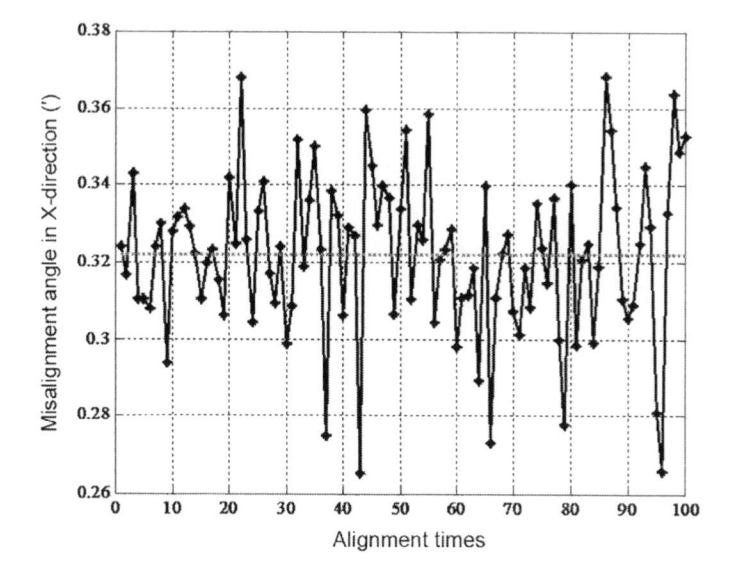

Fig. 4.7 *X*-direction misalignment angle

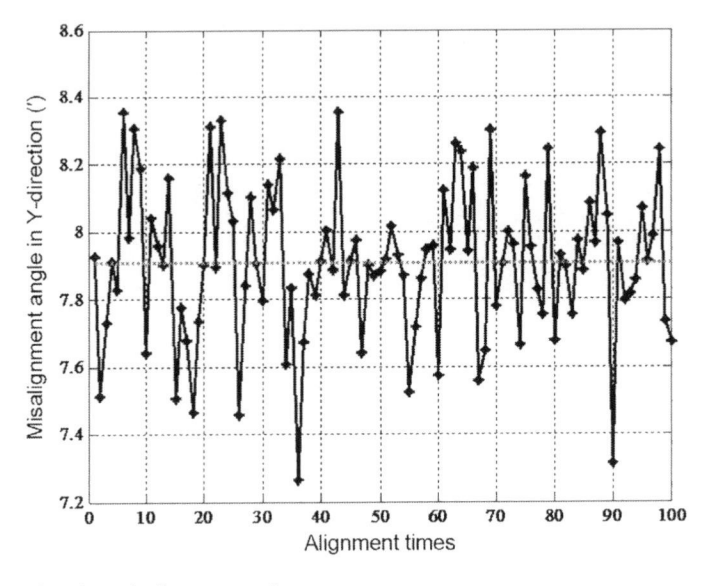

Fig. 4.8 *Y*-direction misalignment angle

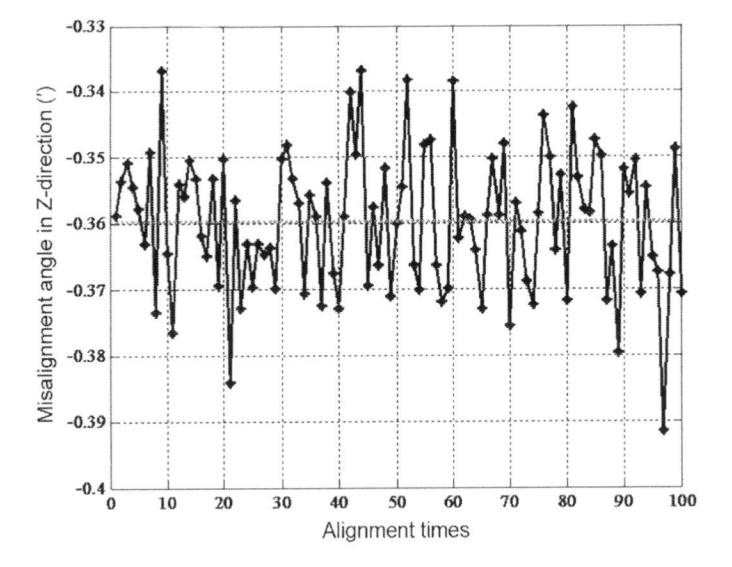

Fig. 4.9 *Z*-direction misalignment angle

of alignment based on inertial system introduced in Sect. 4.3, carry out 100 experiments of simulated alignment. Of these, t_l and t_m are taken as 30 and 150 s respectively. The attitude error angle when alignment completed is shown in Figs. 4.7, 4.8, and 4.9.

The full line in Figs. 4.7, 4.8, and 4.9 shows the values of misalignment angle in each experiment. The dotted line shows the average value of 100 simulations. From Eq. (4.3.7), the calculated theoretical values of misalignment angle in three directions obtained are 0.3250′, 7.8966′, and −0.3664′, respectively, while the average of 100 simulated experiments are 0.3242′, 7.9265′, and −0.3587′, the deviation from the theoretical value are −0.0008′, 0.0299′, and 0.0077′, respectively. The simulation results are the same as the theoretical analysis.

Reference Documentation

1. Wang, Xinlong. 2013. *Initial Alignment of Mobile Base and Stationary Base of Strapdown Inertial Navigation System*. Northwest Industrial University Press.
2. Deng, Zhenglong. 2006. *Inertial Technology*. Harbin Institute of Technology Press.
3. Quan, Wei. 2011. *INS/CNS/GNSS Integrated Navigation Technology*. National Defense Industry Press.
4. Zhong, Xiaoli. 2013. *Research on Initial Alignment Method of Rocket-Borne Strapdown Inertial Navigation System*. Southeast University.
5. Liang, Hao. 2012. *Research on Initial Azimuth Alignment and Orbit Correction Technology*. Harbin Institute of Technology.
6. He, Haiou. 2007. *Research on Initial Alignment Technology of Missile-Borne Strapdown Inertial Navigation System Under the Action of Strong Gust Wind*. Northwest Industrial University.
7. Yi, Zhang. 2012. *Research on Initial Alignment Technology of Shipborne Strapdown Inertial Navigation System*. Harbin Engineering University.
8. Jin, Wang. 2005. *Research on Compass Alignment Method of Strapdown Inertial Navigation System*. Changsha: National University of Defense Technology.
9. Gao, Wei, Yueyang Ben, Qian Li. 2013. *Initial Alignment Technology of Strapdown Inertial Navigation System*. National Defense Industry Press.
10. Darf, Richard C., Robert H. Bishop. 2001. *Modern Control System (Version VIII)*. Translated by Hongwei Xie, Fengxing Zou, Ming Zhang, Pengbo Li, and Qi Li. Higher Education Press.
11. Feng, Peide, Xiudi Mi, etc. 1999. New Path of Alignment of Mobile Base of Inertial Navigation System. *Journal of Chinese Inertial Technology* 9 (4).
12. Ogata, K. 2003. *Modern Control Engineering (Version IV)*. Translated by Boying Lu, Haixun Yu, etc. Publishing House of Electronics Industry.
13. Li, Zigang, Dejun Wan. *Strapdown Inertial Navigation Technology*. China Ship Information Center.
14. Wang, Yongge. 2007. *Realization of MATLAB for Digital Signal Processing*. Science Press.

Chapter 5
INS/GNSS Integrated Navigation Technology

5.1 Introduction

As one type of autonomous navigation system, the inertial navigation does not need to receive any external information. Relying on the data measured by gyroscope and accelerometer, it could solve the motional parameters of position, velocity, and attitude via navigation computer, which is the most important navigation system for the OTV. However, due to the integral principle in solution of inertial navigation, the error of inertial devices will accumulate the navigation error along with time elapses. Therefore, pure INS is unable to meet the requirements of high-precision navigation of long-range- and long-time movement of the OTV.

Satellite navigation is one kind of space-based radio navigation system developed along with space technology on the basis of radio technology. Usually, one generalized concept—Global Positioning System is the collective term for all the satellite navigation positioning systems on orbit. At present, it mainly includes the GPS of the US, Russian GLONASS system, European Galileo System, Chinese BeiDou navigation system (BD-2). The advantages of satellite are of high positioning accuracy, navigation error not cumulative with time elapsing, all-time and all-weather work. However, the satellite navigation system is difficult to provide the attitude information directly, with lower data update rate.

Obviously, INS and GNSS have own respective advantages and weakness. Any type is hard to meet the demands of long-time- and high-performance navigation independently for the OTV. Therefore, the integration of INS and GNSS could have complementary advantages, which is the effective means to realize the high-precision-, high-reliable navigation for the OTV.

© Springer Nature Singapore Pte Ltd. and National Defense Industry Press, Beijing 2018
X. Li and C. Li, *Navigation and Guidance of Orbital Transfer Vehicle*, Navigation: Science and Technology, https://doi.org/10.1007/978-981-10-6334-3_5

5.2 Principle of Satellite Navigation

In satellite navigation positioning, due to the effects of various error sources, the distance values measured do not really reflect the geometric distance between the satellite and navigation receiver, which contains certain error. The satellite navigation measurement distance that contains error is called pseudo-range. It contains the clock errors of the navigation constellation satellite clock and that of the navigation receiver.

Refer to Fig. 5.1. Vector **r** shows the offset vector from the flight vehicle to the navigation satellite. Vector **s** represents the position of navigation satellite corresponding to the coordinate origin, which is calculated by ephemeris data of satellite broadcasting. The vector **r** from satellite to flight vehicle is

$$r = s - u \tag{5.2.1}$$

The amplitude of vector **r** is

$$r = \|s - u\| \tag{5.2.2}$$

The satellite navigation adopts the system of multi-satellites, high orbit, and ranging. It takes distance as the basic observed quantity. Through the receiver mounted on the flight vehicle, measure the time difference τ between the radio wave emitted by the satellite and received by the receiver, multiply the propagation velocity of electromagnetic wave (solving the range), that is

Fig. 5.1 Vector representation of position of flight vehicle

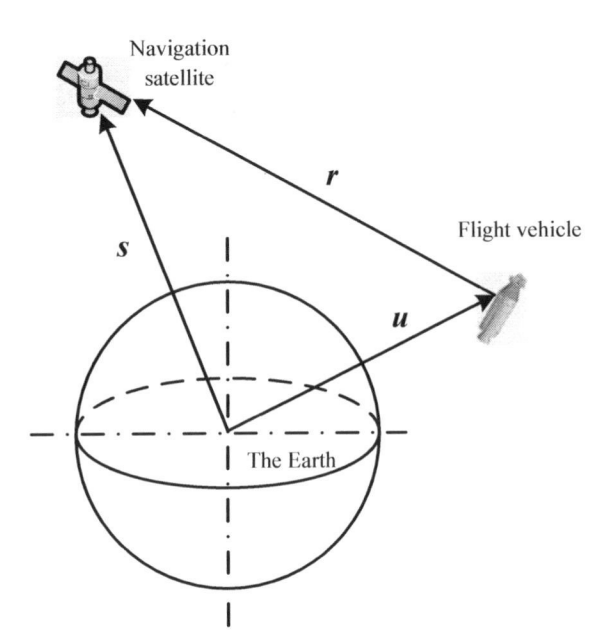

$$r = c \cdot \tau = c(T_u - T_s) \tag{5.2.3}$$

In it, T_u is the system time of signal arrived at the receiver of the user. T_s is the system time of signal leaving the satellite. Satellite navigation usually adopts the atomic time system (JATC). Because the clocks of satellite and the receiver do not synchronize with the system atomic time, there exists clock difference. Given δt is the offset between satellite clock and the system time, t_u is the offset between the clock of receiver and the system time. Then,

$$\rho = c[(T_u + t_u) - (T_s + \delta t)] = c(T_u - T_s) + c(t_u - \delta t) = r + c(t_u - \delta t) \tag{5.2.4}$$

It is evident that the distance observation value ρ contains the error caused by the clock difference of receiver, instead of the real distance r from the receiver to the satellite. It is the pseudo-range observation. Therefore, Eq. (5.2.4) may be rewritten as

$$\rho - c(t_u - \delta t) = \|\mathbf{s} - \mathbf{u}\| \tag{5.2.5}$$

The offset δt between the satellite clock and the system time is composed of the offset deviation and drift. In the following analysis, assumed such offset has been compensated, that is δt is no longer one unknown number. Thus, Eq. (5.2.5) may be recorded as

$$\rho - ct_u = \|\mathbf{s} - \mathbf{u}\| \tag{5.2.6}$$

5.2.1   Principle of Satellite Navigation Pseudo-range Positioning

From the previous analysis, we could know that to determine the position of flight vehicle, the quantities to be solved contain three position quantities and one-time deviation. Carry out pseudo-range measurement of not less than four satellites via the receiver. Then, solve the position of the receiver with the satellite position and pseudo-range measurement provided by navigation message.

From the principle of pseudo-range positioning Eq. (5.2.6) (considering the satellite clock difference), the function relational expression between the measurement quantity and the parameters to be solved is

$$\rho_j = \|\mathbf{s}_j - \mathbf{u}\| + ct_u \tag{5.2.7}$$

In it, the range of j is 1–4 that refers to different satellites. ρ_j is the pseudo measurement value of the j satellite. Equation (5.2.7) may be expanded as the simultaneous equations shown by unknown numbers of x, y, z and t_u,

$$\rho_1 = \sqrt{(x - x_1)^2 + (y - y_1)^2 + (z - z_1)^2} + ct_u \qquad (5.2.8)$$

$$\rho_2 = \sqrt{(x - x_2)^2 + (y - y_2)^2 + (z - z_2)^2} + ct_u \qquad (5.2.9)$$

$$\rho_3 = \sqrt{(x - x_3)^2 + (y - y_3)^2 + (z - z_3)^2} + ct_u \qquad (5.2.10)$$

$$\rho_4 = \sqrt{(x - x_4)^2 + (y - y_4)^2 + (z - z_4)^2} + ct_u \qquad (5.2.11)$$

Here, x_j, y_j, z_j refers to the three-dimensional position of the j satellite.

If we approximately know the position of receiver $(\hat{x}, \hat{y}, \hat{z})$ and the estimated value of time deviation value $\hat{t}_u$, the deviation between the truth pseudo-range and approximate pseudo-range is marked with $(\Delta x, \Delta y, \Delta z, \Delta t_u)$. Expand Eqs. (5.2.8)–(5.2.11) at the place of $(\hat{x}, \hat{y}, \hat{z}, \hat{t}_u)$ according to Taylor's series, the offset $(\Delta x, \Delta y, \Delta z, \Delta t_u)$ is shown by the linear function of known coordinate and pseudo-range measurement.

Record,

$$\Delta \rho_j = \hat{\rho}_j - \rho_j, e_{j1} = \frac{x_j - \hat{x}}{\hat{r}_j}, e_{j2} = \frac{y_j - \hat{y}}{\hat{r}_j}, e_{j3} = \frac{z_j - \hat{z}}{\hat{r}_j} \qquad (5.2.12)$$

Expand with Taylor's series, and obtain,

$$\Delta \rho_j = e_{j1} \Delta x + e_{j2} \Delta y + e_{j3} \Delta z - c \Delta t_u$$

Since there are four unknown quantities $\Delta x, \Delta y, \Delta z$ and Δt_u, measure the range of four satellites and solve. These known quantities could be solved by the following simultaneous linear equations:

$$\begin{aligned}
\Delta \rho_1 &= e_{11} \Delta x + e_{12} \Delta y + e_{13} \Delta z - c \Delta t_u \\
\Delta \rho_2 &= e_{21} \Delta x + e_{22} \Delta y + e_{23} \Delta z - c \Delta t_u \\
\Delta \rho_3 &= e_{31} \Delta x + e_{32} \Delta y + e_{33} \Delta z - c \Delta t_u \\
\Delta \rho_4 &= e_{41} \Delta x + e_{42} \Delta y + e_{43} \Delta z - c \Delta t_u
\end{aligned} \qquad (5.2.13)$$

Equation (5.2.13) may be written in the form of matrix with the following definitions:

$$\Delta \rho = \begin{bmatrix} \Delta \rho_1 \\ \Delta \rho_2 \\ \Delta \rho_3 \\ \Delta \rho_4 \end{bmatrix}, H = \begin{bmatrix} e_{11} & e_{12} & e_{13} & -1 \\ e_{21} & e_{22} & e_{23} & -1 \\ e_{31} & e_{32} & e_{33} & -1 \\ e_{41} & e_{42} & e_{43} & -1 \end{bmatrix}, \Delta X = \begin{bmatrix} \Delta x \\ \Delta y \\ \Delta z \\ c \Delta t_u \end{bmatrix}$$

At last, obtain,

$$\Delta\rho = H\Delta X \tag{5.2.14}$$

Its solution is

$$\Delta X = H^{-1}\Delta\rho \tag{5.2.15}$$

Once the known quantity is solved, use Eq. (5.2.14) to calculate the coordinates x, y, and z of the user and the clock skew t_u of the receiver. Such linear method is feasible as long as the shift $(\Delta x, \Delta y, \Delta z)$ is near to the linear point. If the shift is certain to exceed the accepted value, iterate the above-mentioned process, that is to take the calculated point x, y, and z as the new estimated value to take the place of $\hat{\rho}$.

5.2.2 Principle of Determining Velocity of Satellite Navigation

Besides providing the coordinates of three positions and precise times for flight vehicle, satellite navigation also provides velocity of the flight vehicle. As for many modern navigation receivers, estimate the Doppler frequency of satellite signal received precisely by processing the phase measurement value of the carrier, so as to measure the velocity. On the antenna of receiver, the frequency f_R received is approximately shown by traditional Doppler equation as follows:

$$f_R = f_T\left(1 - \frac{v_r \cdot e}{c}\right) \tag{5.2.16}$$

In it, f_T is the frequency of satellite signal; v_r is the relative velocity vector between satellite and the flight vehicle. e is the unit vector of straight line of flight vehicle pointing at satellite. c is the light velocity, vector v_r is the velocity difference into geocentric inertial coordinate system.

$$v_r = v - \dot{u} \tag{5.2.17}$$

In it, v is the velocity of satellite; $\dot{u}$ is the velocity of flight vehicle.
As for the j satellite, put Eq. (5.2.18) into Eq. (5.2.17), obtain

$$f_{Rj} = f_{Tj}\left\{1 - \frac{1}{c}\left[(v_j - \dot{u}) \cdot e\right]\right\} \tag{5.2.18}$$

Obtain the actual emission frequency of satellite from the receiver, that is,

$$f_{Tj} = f_0 + \Delta f_{Tj} \tag{5.2.19}$$

In it, f_0 is the nominal emission frequency of satellite, Δf_{Tj} is the correction value determined by updated navigation message.

As for the j satellite, the measurement estimated value of the frequency of signal received is recorded as f_j. The clock drift error f_j and f_{Rj} have the following relations:

$$f_{Rj} = f_j(1 + i_u) \tag{5.2.20}$$

Put Eq. (5.2.21) into Eq. (5.2.19) and obtain,

$$\frac{c(f_j - f_{Tj})}{f_{Tj}} + v_{jx}e_{j1} + v_{jy}e_{j2} + v_{jz}e_{j3} = \dot{x}e_{j1} + \dot{y}e_{j2} + \dot{z}e_{j3} - \frac{cf_j i_u}{f_{Tj}} \tag{5.2.21}$$

Here, $v_j = (v_{jx} \quad v_{jy} \quad v_{jz})$, $e_j = (e_{j1} \quad e_{j2} \quad e_{j3})$, $\dot{u} = (\dot{x}, \dot{y}, \dot{z})$. Introduce new variable d_j, its definition is

$$d_j = \frac{c(f_j - f_{Tj})}{f_{Tj}} + v_{jx}e_{j1} + v_{jy}e_{j2} + v_{jz}e_{j3} \tag{5.2.22}$$

Commonly, f_j/f_{Tj} is very close to 1. After simplifying, obtain from Eq. (5.2.22),

$$d_j = \dot{x}e_{j1} + \dot{y}e_{j2} + \dot{z}e_{j3} - ci_u \tag{5.2.23}$$

Thus, there are four known numbers $\dot{x}, \dot{y}, \dot{z}$ and i_u, which are solved by measuring four satellites. Apply matrix algorithm to solve the simultaneous equations to calculate the known quantity. These matrixes/vectors are shown as

$$d = \begin{bmatrix} d_1 \\ d_2 \\ d_3 \\ d_4 \end{bmatrix}, H = \begin{bmatrix} e_{11} & e_{12} & e_{13} & -1 \\ e_{21} & e_{22} & e_{23} & -1 \\ e_{31} & e_{32} & e_{33} & -1 \\ e_{41} & e_{42} & e_{43} & -1 \end{bmatrix}, g = \begin{bmatrix} \dot{x} \\ \dot{y} \\ \dot{z} \\ ci_u \end{bmatrix}$$

Record $d = Hg$, the solutions of velocity and time drift rate are, $g = H^{-1}d$.

The frequency estimations in velocity formula are obtained from phase measurement, which is affected by the errors of measurement noise and multipath. Furthermore, the calculation of velocity of flight vehicle is determined by the accuracy of vehicle position and the correct control of ephemeris and velocity of satellite.

5.2.3 Principle of Satellite Navigation Attitude Determination

Attitude measurement of satellite navigation is the technology developed in last 20 years. Its basic principle is to measure the projection of baseline vector formed by antenna on the line vector of navigation satellite by laying multi-antennas. Refer to Fig. 5.2. k1 and k2 are the two navigation antennas that are separated in range and mounted on the flight vehicle. Measure the phase difference of multi-satellites on the k1 and k2 antennas, calculate and solve the baseline vectors. The double or multi-baseline measurement system formed by three or multi-antennas could measure three attitude angles of the measuring carrier. The attitude observation equation established in such mode is called single difference equation.

In engineering practice, to cancel clock difference between the receivers, reduce the linear deviation and improve the accuracy of attitude determination, the double difference equation could be obtained by the difference of two single difference equations. The attitude determination principle is the same as the single difference equation, which has one more observation satellite. Refer to Fig. 5.3.

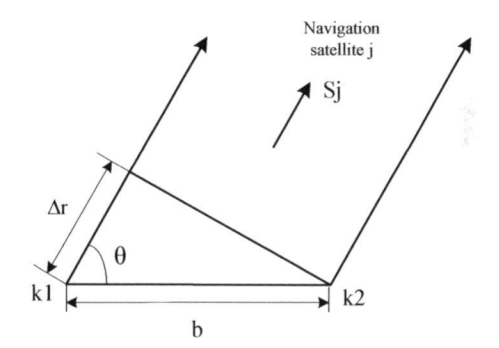

Fig. 5.2 Schematic diagram of single difference equation

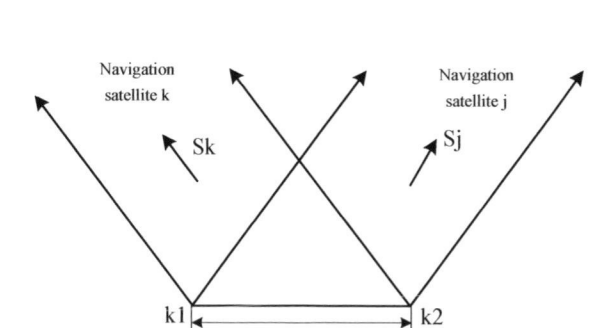

Fig. 5.3 Schematic diagram of double difference equation

5.3   Principle of INS/GNSS Integrated Navigation System

5.3.1   Combination Mode of INS/GNSS Integrated Navigation

The INS/GNSS navigation system could be integrated into different modes according to the different requirements of applications. According to the depth of integration, the integrated navigation system is roughly classified into the loose integration, tight integration, and deep integration.

1. Loose Integration

Main characteristics of loose integration are that the navigation receiver and inertial navigation system work independently. The role of integration is only shown by the navigation receiver aiding the INS. The block diagram of principle is shown in Fig. 5.4. The difference between the position and velocity information transmitted by navigation receiver and INS are taken as the observation quantity, to estimate the error of INS through combined Kalman filter. Then, correct the INS.

The work in loose integration is simpler, easy to realize in engineering, and the two systems work independently, which provides certain redundancy for the navigation information.

2. Tight Integration

Compared to the loose integration, the basic mode of tight integration is the combination of pseudo-range and pseudo-range rate. Its principle is shown in Fig. 5.5. Solve the pseudo-range ρ_I and pseudo-range rate $\dot{\rho}_I$ that correspond to the INS position and velocity with the ephemeris data provided by navigation receiver and the position and velocity given by the INS. Compare the ρ_I and $\dot{\rho}_I$ with the ρ_I and $\dot{\rho}_G$ measured by navigation receiver as the observation quantity. Estimate the error quantity of INS and navigation receiver via combined Kalman filters, then, correct the two systems. Since it is easy to set up modeling for the range error of the navigation receiver, it could be expanded as state, and estimated by combined filter, so as to correct the navigation receiver.

The integration mode of pseudo-range and pseudo-range rate commonly has higher reliability than the integration of position and velocity. In tight integration,

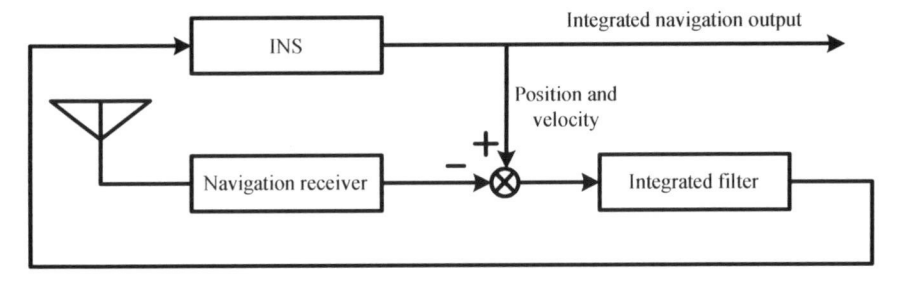

Fig. 5.4 Integration of position and velocity

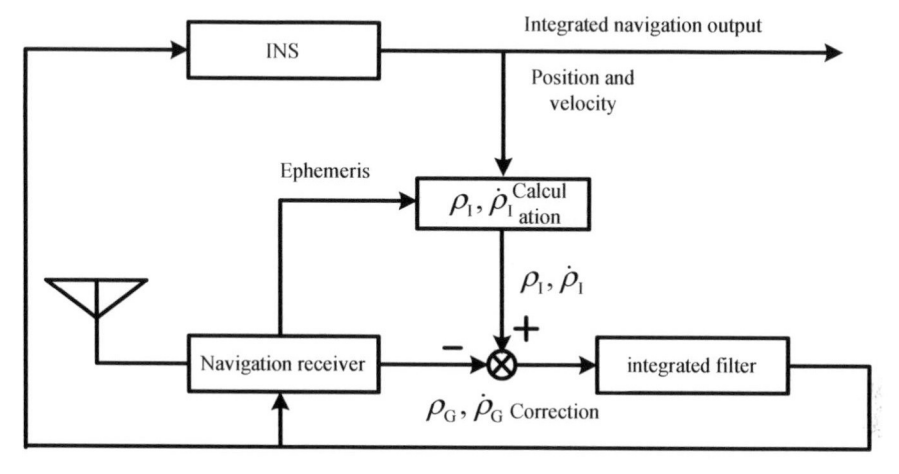

Fig. 5.5 Functional block diagram of pseudo-range and pseudo-range rate integration

the navigation receiver only provides ephemeris data, pseudo-range and pseudo-range rate, which has omitted the part of navigation calculation.

3. Deep Integration

The deep integration technology was put forward at the mid- and late 1990s, which is an important typical feature of American next-generation military navigation system. As one concept and connotation, the core of the deep integration technology is to assist loop tracking of the receiver by the navigation results of GNSS/INS integration, and take the output of the devices concerned as the observation quantity directly. One integrated filter could fulfill the error estimation of combined navigation and receiver, which separates the deep integration from the tight integration characterized by pseudo-range and pseudo-range rate.

Compared with the loose integration and tight integration, the deep integration could improve the working performance of navigation receiver, and increase the adaptability of navigation receiver for high-dynamic motional carrier. At present, the research institutions and personnel, both at home and abroad, are studying multi-aspects of deep integration including the specific framework system, filtering method, and hardware platform.

5.3.2   Fundamentals of INS/GNSS Integrated Navigation

The fundamentals of INS-/GNSS- integrated navigation is to take the error equation of INS and GNSS system as the system state equation, and take the information sent by the two systems as the measurement quantity, to realize high precise integrated navigation by Kalman filter. Refer to Fig. 5.6.

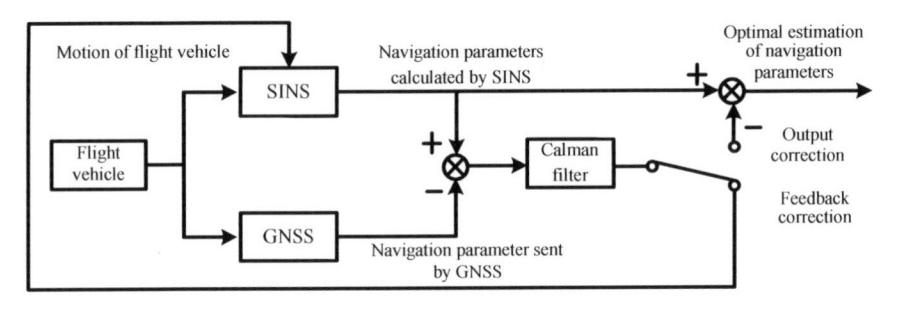

Fig. 5.6 Schematic diagram of indirect filtering

From Fig. 5.6, we can know that after we obtain the estimation value of Kalman filter, i.e., the navigation error, there are two methods, one is the output correction method and the other is the feedback correction method.

The Output Correction Method is to correct the navigation parameters transmitted by INS with the estimated value $\Delta \hat{X}_I$ of the INS parameter error, and obtain the estimated value $\hat{X}$ of the navigation parameters of the integrated navigation system (the system navigation parameters corrected), that is, $\hat{X} = X_I - \Delta \hat{X}_I$. The output correction method improves the accuracy of navigation positioning by correcting the system output directly. Its advantage is that the INS and filter work independently, with good system stability, and easy realization in engineering practice.

The feedback correction method is to feed the estimated value $\Delta \hat{X}_I$ of the INS navigation parameter error ΔX_I to the INS and correct the error state, that is, to correct the velocity, position, and strapdown matrix with error in the mechanics equation. Carry out next navigation solution by taking the corrected parameters as the initial values. Whereas, the error of inertial devices is the direct cause of decrease of navigation precision of the INS, compensate the output of inertial devices directly with the estimated values of gyroscope drift and zero offset of the accelerometer. This is also one application of feedback correction. Under which, the navigation parameters transmitted by INS is the output of the integrated navigation system.

5.4 Design of INS/GNSS Integrated Navigation System

5.4.1 Design of Loose Integration Navigation System

The loose integration is the integration mode that is easy to be realized. The INS and satellite navigation receiver work independently. The difference value of position and velocity information transmitted by navigation receiver and INS is used for observation quantity, through Kalman filtering, to estimate the error of the INS. Then, correct the INS system. Since the Kalman filtering describes the random linear system with state equation and measurement equation, it needs to derive the system model before applying the Kalman filtering.

1. Mathematic model of integrated navigation system—State Equation

The mathematical model of integrated navigation system refers to the system state equation and measurement equation in Fig. 5.4.

When the integrated navigation system adopts linear Kalman filter(LKF), it takes the error of navigation output parameter of the INS as the state. The navigation output parameters of INS system have nine, three error angles of inertial navigation platform, three velocity errors, and three position errors. It takes the launching inertial system as the navigation coordinate system, in combination with the error vector equation expression of the INS, assuming the earth as the rotational ellipsoid, the error scalar equation of INS could be given.

(1) Platform Error Angle Equation

$$\begin{bmatrix} \dot{\phi}_x \\ \dot{\phi}_y \\ \dot{\phi}_z \end{bmatrix} = -C_b^n \begin{bmatrix} \varepsilon_x + W_{\varepsilon_x} \\ \varepsilon_y + W_{\varepsilon_y} \\ \varepsilon_z + W_{\varepsilon_z} \end{bmatrix} \tag{5.4.1}$$

(2) Velocity Error Equation

$$\begin{bmatrix} \delta\dot{V}_x \\ \delta\dot{V}_y \\ \delta\dot{V}_z \end{bmatrix} = F_g \begin{bmatrix} \delta x \\ \delta y \\ \delta z \end{bmatrix} + F_f \begin{bmatrix} \phi_x \\ \phi_y \\ \phi_z \end{bmatrix} + C_b^n \begin{bmatrix} \nabla_x + W_{\nabla x} \\ \nabla_y + W_{\nabla y} \\ \nabla_z + W_{\nabla z} \end{bmatrix} \tag{5.4.2}$$

In it, $(\delta V_x, \delta V_y, \delta V_z)$ is the velocity error of flight vehicle in three axle direction of the inertial coordinate system of launch point. $(\delta x, \delta y, \delta z)$ is the position errors of the flight vehicle in three axle directions of inertial coordinate system of launch point. F_g is the gravitational term and $F_f = (C_b^n \cdot f^b)^k$ is the anti-symmetric matrix formed by $C_b^n \cdot f^b$.

(3) Position Error Equation

$$\begin{bmatrix} \delta\dot{x} \\ \delta\dot{y} \\ \delta\dot{z} \end{bmatrix} = \begin{bmatrix} 1 & 0 & 0 \\ 0 & 1 & 0 \\ 0 & 0 & 1 \end{bmatrix} \begin{bmatrix} \delta V_x \\ \delta V_y \\ \delta V_z \end{bmatrix} \tag{5.4.3}$$

(4) Error of Inertial devices

Similar to this chapter, the error of inertial devices is simplified as random constant in unity for consideration.

① Gyroscope drift error model

$$\dot{\varepsilon}_x = 0, \dot{\varepsilon}_y = 0, \dot{\varepsilon}_z = 0 \tag{5.4.4}$$

② Accelerometer error model

$$\dot{\nabla}_x = 0, \dot{\nabla}_y = 0, \dot{\nabla}_z = 0 \tag{5.4.5}$$

Merge the six states of error of inertial devices with the error of nine states of navigation output parameters of INS, obtain the 15-dimensional system state equation as

$$\dot{X}(t) = F_I(t)X(t) + G_I(t)W(t) \tag{5.4.6}$$

In it, the state vector $X(t)$ and the system noise vector $W(t)$ are,

$$X(t) = \left[\phi_x, \phi_y, \phi_z, \delta V_x, \delta V_y, \delta V_z, \delta x, \delta y, \delta z, \varepsilon_x, \varepsilon_y, \varepsilon_z, \nabla_x, \nabla_y, \nabla_z\right]^{\mathrm{T}} \tag{5.4.7}$$

$$W(t) = \left[W_{\varepsilon_x}, W_{\varepsilon_y}, W_{\varepsilon_z}, W_{\nabla_x}, W_{\nabla_y}, W_{\nabla_z}\right]^{\mathrm{T}} \tag{5.4.8}$$

From the previous analysis, we could know that the system state coefficient matrix $F_I(t)$ and the error coefficient matrix $G_I(t)$ are the respective,

$$F_I(t) = \begin{bmatrix} 0_{3\times3} & 0_{3\times3} & 0_{3\times3} & -C_b^n & 0_{3\times3} \\ F_f & 0_{3\times3} & F_g & 0_{3\times3} & C_b^n \\ 0_{3\times3} & I_{3\times3} & 0_{3\times3} & 0_{3\times3} & 0_{3\times3} \\ 0_{3\times3} & 0_{3\times3} & 0_{3\times3} & 0_{3\times3} & 0_{3\times3} \\ 0_{3\times3} & 0_{3\times3} & 0_{3\times3} & 0_{3\times3} & 0_{3\times3} \end{bmatrix}_{15\times15} \tag{5.4.9}$$

$$G_I(t) = \begin{bmatrix} -C_b^n & 0_{3\times3} \\ 0_{3\times3} & C_b^n \\ 0_{3\times3} & 0_{3\times3} \\ 0_{3\times3} & 0_{3\times3} \\ 0_{3\times3} & 0_{3\times3} \end{bmatrix}_{15\times6} \tag{5.4.10}$$

2. Mathematical model of integrated navigation system—measurement equation

In the integrated modes of position and velocity (the combination relations refers to Fig. 5.1), Its observation quantity is obtained by the velocity and position information solved by navigation calculation minus that output by navigation receiver. At this moment, the measurement equation is

$$Z(t) = \mathrm{INS}_{S,V} - \mathrm{GNSS}_{S,V} = \begin{bmatrix} x_I - x_G \\ y_I - y_G \\ z_I - z_G \\ v_{Ix} - v_{Gx} \\ v_{Iy} - v_{Gy} \\ v_{Iz} - v_{Gz} \end{bmatrix} = H(t)X(t) + V(t) \tag{5.4.11}$$

In it, (x_I, y_I, z_I) are the three axis components in launching inertial system of the carrier position obtained by calculating inertial navigation. (v_{Ix}, v_{Iy}, v_{Iz}) are the three axis components of carrier velocity in launching inertial system obtained by calculating inertial navigation. (x_G, y_G, z_G) are the three axis components of carrier position in launching inertial system transmitted by navigation receiver. (v_{Gx}, v_{Gy}, v_{Gz}) are the three axis components of carrier velocity in launching inertial system transmitted by navigation receiver.

From Eq. (5.4.11) we can know that the measurement equation shall need the position and velocity solved by satellite navigation. Thus, the loosely integrated navigation system shall observe at least four satellites.

After obtaining state equation and measurement equation, discretize the equations, that is, process with Kalman filter.

5.4.2 Design of Tight Integrated Navigation System

The characteristics of tight integrated navigation system are of simple integrated plan and easy to realize. However, when the flight vehicle carries out high-dynamic maneuvers or if the navigation receiver is unable to work for long time because of the environmental interference, the system accuracy will be reduced sharply and along with the time increasing, the reliability and anti-interference capability are poor. Corresponding to the loosely integrated mode, the navigation receiver in tight integration could only provide the original, direct ephemeris and pseudo-range and pseudo-range data, which do not need navigation solution. The information are used for correcting INS via Kalman filtering, for the system to obtain better navigation performance.

1. Mathematical model of integrated navigation system

It adopts the schematic diagram shown in Fig. 5.5, in which receiver provides pseudo-range and pseudo-range rate. The main error term is the clock error. The modeling rule is clear. The state of integrated navigation filter consists of two parts, one is the error state of the INS, its state equation reference type (5.8), and the other part is the added error state of navigation receiver. The error state of GPS receiver is the colored noise, which is usually two, one is the distance related to equivalent clock error δt_u, and the other is the distance rate δt_{ru} related to the equivalent clock frequency error.

(1) State Equation of the System

Expand the distance related to equivalent clock error and the distance rate related to equivalent clock frequency error of the navigation receiver into system state, that is

$$X_G = [\delta t_u \quad \delta t_{ru}]^{\mathrm{T}} \tag{5.4.12}$$

Its differential equation is

$$\begin{aligned} \dot{\delta t}_u &= \delta t_u + w_{tu} \\ \dot{\delta t}_{ru} &= -\beta_{tru}\delta t_{ru} + w_{tru} \end{aligned} \tag{5.4.13}$$

That is,

$$\dot{X}_G(t) = F_G(t)X_G(t) + G_G(t)W_G(t) \tag{5.4.14}$$

In it,

$$F_G(t) = \begin{bmatrix} 0 & 1 \\ 0 & -\beta_{tru} \end{bmatrix} \tag{5.4.15}$$

$$G_G(t) = \begin{bmatrix} 1 & 0 \\ 0 & 1 \end{bmatrix} \tag{5.4.16}$$

Combine Eqs. (5.4.6) and (5.4.19), obtain the system state equation (17 dimensions) of the pseudo-range and pseudo-range rate as

$$\begin{bmatrix} \dot{X}_I(t) \\ \hline \dot{X}_G(t) \end{bmatrix} = \begin{bmatrix} F_I(t) & 0 \\ \hline 0 & F_G(t) \end{bmatrix} \begin{bmatrix} X_I(t) \\ \hline X_G(t) \end{bmatrix} + \begin{bmatrix} G_I(t) & 0 \\ \hline 0 & G_G(t) \end{bmatrix} \begin{bmatrix} W_I(t) \\ \hline W_G(t) \end{bmatrix} \tag{5.4.17}$$

That is,

$$\dot{X}(t) = F(t)X(t) + G(t)W(t) \tag{5.4.18}$$

(2) System measurement equation

Assume x, y, and z are the components of three axles of the true carrier position in launching inertial system. The x_I, y_I and z_I are the three axis components of carrier position information in launching inertial system obtained by inertial navigation calculation. The x_{si}, y_{si} and z_{si} are the three axis components of navigation satellite in launching inertial system, obtain the pseudo-range (calculated pseudo-range) between the carrier and satellite ρ_{Ii} as

$$\rho_{Ii} = \left[(x_I - x_{si})^2 + (y_I - y_{si})^2 + (z_I - z_{si})^2 \right]^{\frac{1}{2}} \tag{5.4.19}$$

Expand the above-mentioned formula into Taylor's series corresponding to the true projection x, y, and z and omit the higher order term. We obtain,

$$\rho_{li} = \rho_i + \frac{\partial \rho_{li}}{\partial x} \delta x + \frac{\partial \rho_{li}}{\partial y} \delta y + \frac{\partial \rho_{li}}{\partial z} \delta z \qquad (5.4.20)$$

In it, $\rho_i = \left[(x - x_{si})^2 + (y - y_{si})^2 + (z - z_{si})^2 \right]^{\frac{1}{2}}$, $\delta x = x_I - x$, $\delta y = y_I - y$, $\delta z = z_I - z$, are the position error component of inertial navigation calculation. Let $\frac{\partial \rho_{li}}{\partial x} = \frac{x - x_{si}}{\rho_i} = e_{i1}$, $\frac{\partial \rho_{li}}{\partial y} = \frac{y - y_{si}}{\rho_i} = e_{i2}$, $\frac{\partial \rho_{li}}{\partial z} = \frac{z - z_{si}}{\rho_i} = e_{i3}$, the pseudo-range ρ_{Gi} between the carrier and navigation satellite measured by navigation receiver could be shown as

$$\rho_{Gi} = \rho_i + \delta t_u + v_{\rho i} \qquad (5.4.21)$$

where, $v_{\rho i}$ is the noise of receiver, then, the measurement equation of pseudo-range is

$$\delta \rho_i = \rho_{li} - \rho_{Gi} = e_{i1} \delta x + e_{i2} \delta y + e_{i3} \delta z - \delta t_u - v_{\rho i} \qquad (5.4.22)$$

The pseudo-range rate $\dot{\rho}_{li}$ at the position corresponding to inertial navigation is

$$\dot{\rho}_{li} = [(x_I - x_{si})(\dot{x}_I - \dot{x}_{si}) + (y_I - y_{si})(\dot{y}_I - \dot{y}_{si}) + (z_I - z_{si})(\dot{z}_I - \dot{z}_{si})]/\rho_{li} \quad (5.4.23)$$

Expand $\dot{\rho}_{li}$ in Taylor's series at the place of $(x, y, z, \dot{x}, \dot{y}, \dot{z})$, and omit the higher order term. We obtain,

$$\dot{\rho}_{li} = \dot{\rho}_i + \frac{\partial \dot{\rho}_{li}}{\partial x} \delta x + \frac{\partial \dot{\rho}_{li}}{\partial y} \delta y + \frac{\partial \dot{\rho}_{li}}{\partial z} \delta z + \frac{\partial \dot{\rho}_{li}}{\partial \dot{x}} \delta \dot{x} + \frac{\partial \dot{\rho}_{li}}{\partial \dot{y}} \delta \dot{y} + \frac{\partial \dot{\rho}_{li}}{\partial \dot{z}} \delta \dot{z} \qquad (5.4.24)$$

$$\frac{\partial \dot{\rho}_{li}}{\partial x} = \frac{\dot{x}_I - \dot{x}_{si}}{\rho_{li}} - \frac{\dot{\rho}_{li}(x_I - x_{si})}{\rho_{li}^2} = g_{i1} \qquad (5.4.25)$$

In such manner, we obtain,

$$\frac{\partial \dot{\rho}_{li}}{\partial y} = \frac{\dot{y}_I - \dot{y}_{si}}{\rho_{li}} - \frac{\dot{\rho}_{li}(y_I - y_{si})}{\rho_{li}^2} = g_{i2}, \quad \frac{\partial \dot{\rho}_{li}}{\partial z} = \frac{\dot{z}_I - \dot{z}_{si}}{\rho_{li}} - \frac{\dot{\rho}_{li}(z_I - z_{si})}{\rho_{li}^2} = g_{i3}$$

$$\frac{\partial \dot{\rho}_{li}}{\partial \dot{x}} = e_{i1}, \quad \frac{\partial \dot{\rho}_{li}}{\partial \dot{y}} = e_{i2}, \quad \frac{\partial \dot{\rho}_{li}}{\partial \dot{z}} = e_{i3}$$

$$(5.4.26)$$

The pseudo-range rate $\dot{\rho}_{Gi}$ between the carrier and navigation measured by navigation receiver may be shown as

$$\dot{\rho}_{Gi} = \dot{\rho}_i + \delta t_{ru} + v_{\dot{\rho} i} \qquad (5.4.27)$$

The measurement equation to obtain the pseudo-range rate is

$$
\delta\dot{\rho}_i = \dot{\rho}_{li} - \dot{\rho}_{Gi} = \frac{\partial\dot{\rho}_{li}}{\partial x}\delta x + \frac{\partial\dot{\rho}_{li}}{\partial y}\delta y + \frac{\partial\dot{\rho}_{li}}{\partial z}\delta z + \frac{\partial\dot{\rho}_{li}}{\partial\dot{x}}\delta\dot{x} + \frac{\partial\dot{\rho}_{li}}{\partial\dot{y}}\delta\dot{y} + \frac{\partial\dot{\rho}_{li}}{\partial\dot{z}}\delta\dot{z}
$$
$$
- \delta t_{ru} - v_{\rho i} = g_{i1}\delta x + g_{i2}\delta y + g_{i3}\delta z + e_{i1}\delta\dot{x} + e_{i2}\delta\dot{y} + e_{i3}\delta\dot{z} - \delta t_{ru} - v_{\rho i}
$$

$$(5.4.28)$$

If we take n visible satellites with good geometric positions, the measurement equation of forming the pseudo-range and pseudo-range rate integrated navigation system is

$$
Z = \begin{bmatrix} \delta\rho_1 \\ \delta\dot{\rho}_1 \\ \vdots \\ \delta\rho_n \\ \delta\dot{\rho}_n \end{bmatrix} = \begin{bmatrix} 0_{1\times3} & 0_{1\times3} & e_{1\times3} & 0_{1\times3} & 0_{1\times3} & 1 & 0 \\ 0_{1\times3} & e_{1\times3} & g_{1\times3} & 0_{1\times3} & 0_{1\times3} & 0 & 1 \\ & & \cdots & & & & \\ 0_{1\times3} & 0_{1\times3} & e_{1\times3} & 0_{1\times3} & 0_{1\times3} & 1 & 0 \\ 0_{1\times3} & e_{1\times3} & g_{1\times3} & 0_{1\times3} & 0_{1\times3} & 0 & 1 \end{bmatrix} \qquad (5.4.29)
$$

In it, $e_{1\times3} = [e_{i1} \quad e_{i2} \quad e_{i3}], g_{1\times3} = [g_{i1} \quad g_{i2} \quad g_{i3}]$.

From Eq. (5.4.29) we can know, the measurement equation only needs the pseudo-range and pseudo-range rate measured by navigation receiver, and does not need to calculate the velocity and position of the flight vehicle. Because the system shall estimate the error of position and velocity of the inertial navigation, to guarantee the normal operation of tight integrated navigation system, at least three satellites are needed for observation. Compared with loose integrated mode, the number of satellites observed is reduced, which improves the reliability of the system.

The discretization of the state equation and measurement equation obtained shall be processed by Kalman filter.

5.5 Analysis of Simulation Results

The simulation takes the international Ellipsoid in 1975 as the Earth reference ellipsoid model. The major semi-axis is 6,378,140 m, the oblateness is 1/298.57, and the geocentric gravitational constant is $3,986,005 \times 10^8 \mathrm{m}^3/\mathrm{s}^2$.

The navigation coordinate system chooses the launching inertial system. First, design the trajectory of the flight vehicle. Assume the longitude of launch point of flight vehicle is 135°, the latitude is 45°, elevation height is 10 m and the launch azimuth is 45°. Select one flight section of the flight vehicle for simulation. The position of the start point of such section in launching inertial system is $[2,924,004, -637,984,180,908]$ m ,the velocity is $[6138, -3471, -152]$ m/s, the flight time is 2000s. The sustainer motor of the flight vehicle is at shutdown state, only the attitude motor generates the designated attitude change, the corresponding flight trajectories refer to Figs. 5.7, 5.8, 5.9, 5.10, 5.11, 5.12, 5.13, 5.14 and 5.15.

In terms of the established flight trajectory, take the constant drift of micro-gyroscope as 0.02°/h, the mean square root of white noise is 0.01°/h; the zero offset of micro-accelerometer is 0.001 g, the mean square roof of white noise is 0.0001 g; the solving cycle of inertial navigation is 0.1 s, the simulation results obtained under the function of inertial navigation refer to Figs. 5.16, 5.17, 5.18, 5.19, 5.20, 5.21, 5.22, 5.23 and 5.24.

From the simulation results we can know, the navigation error of inertial navigation is divergent along with time (in particular the position and velocity) elapses, which could not meet the demands of long-term high-precision navigation of flight vehicle. It should be integrated with other navigation systems.

Fig. 5.7 Curve of yaw angle change

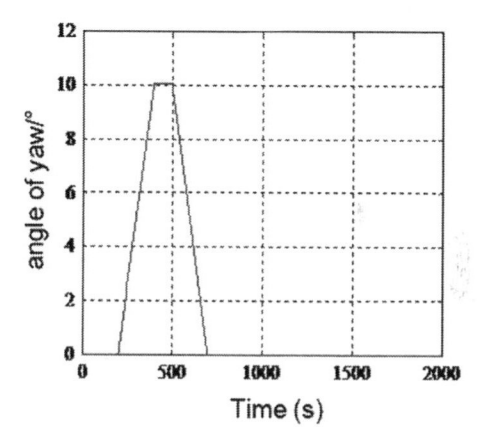

Fig. 5.8 Curve of pitch angle change

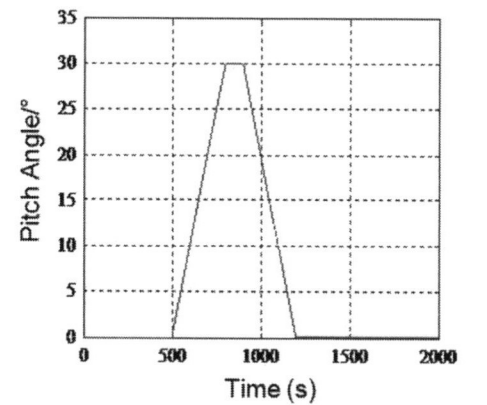

Fig. 5.9 Curve of rolling
angle change

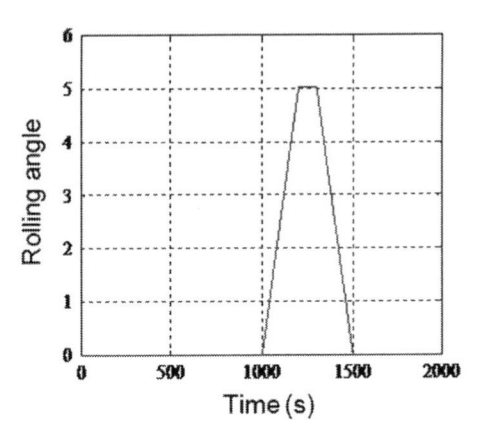

Fig. 5.10 Curve of x-axis
velocity change

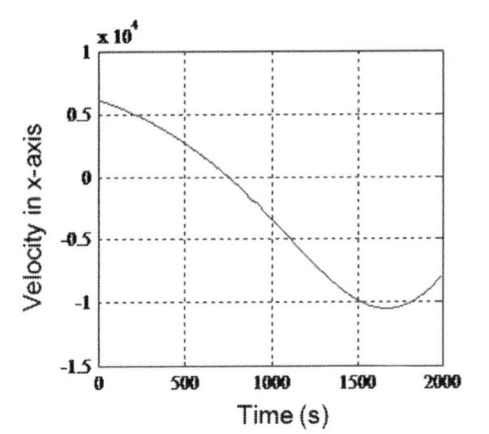

Fig. 5.11 Curve of y-axis
velocity change

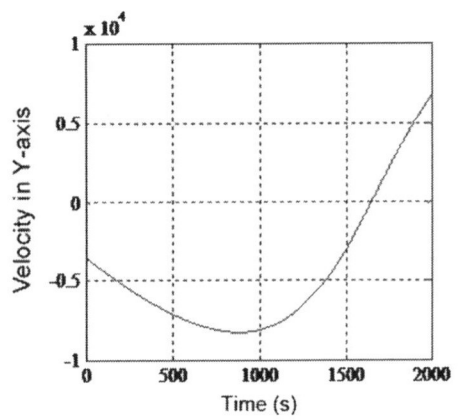

Fig. 5.12 Cruve of z-axis
velocity change

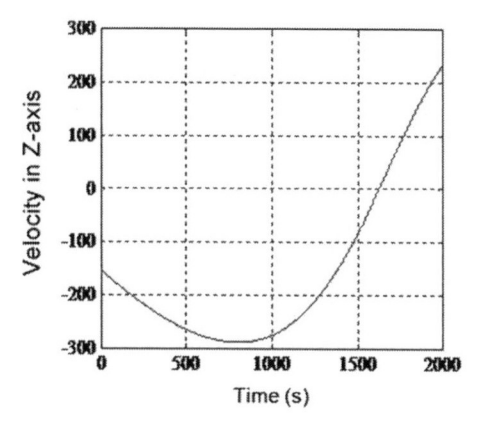

Fig. 5.13 Curve of x-axis
position change

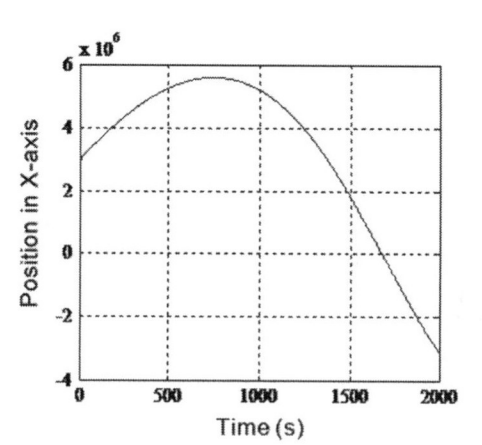

Fig. 5.14 Curve of y-axis
position change

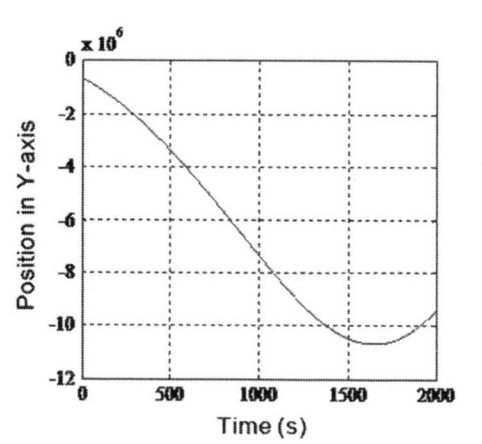

Fig. 5.15 Curve of z-axis
position change

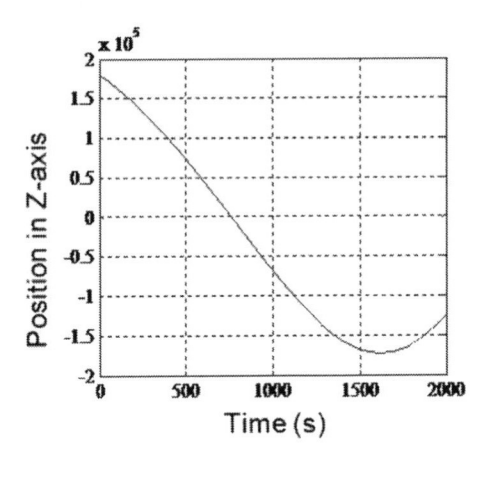

Fig. 5.16 Curve of inertial
navigation yaw deviation

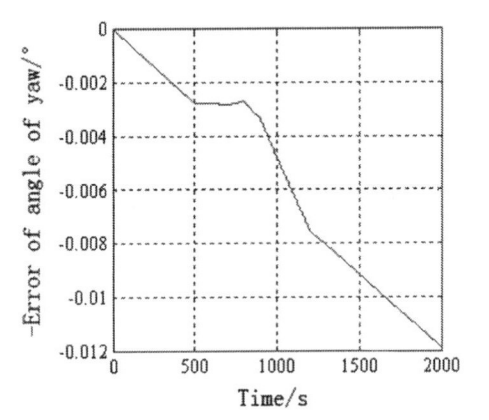

Fig. 5.17 Curve of inertial
navigation pitch deviation

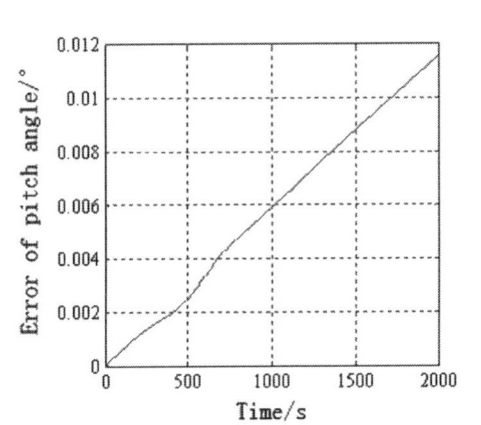

Fig. 5.18 Curve of inertial
navigation rolling angle
deviation

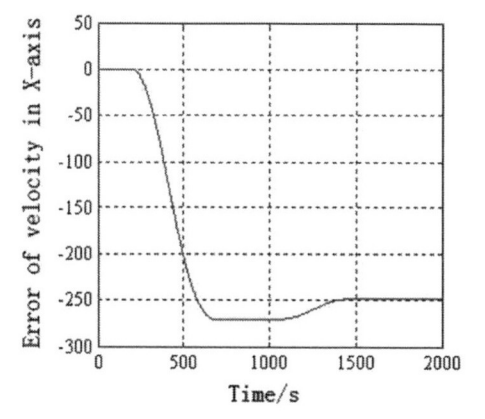

Fig. 5.19 Curve of inertial
navigation x-axis velocity
deviation

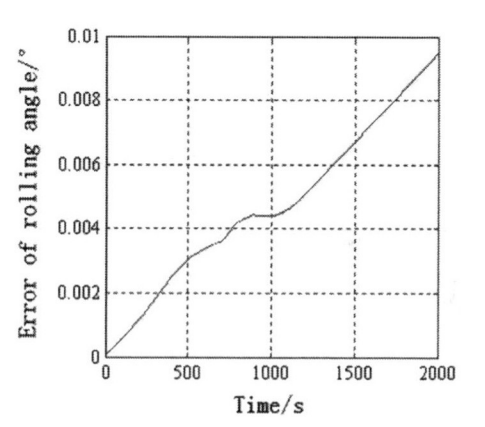

Fig. 5.20 Curve of inertial
navigation y-axis velocity
deviation

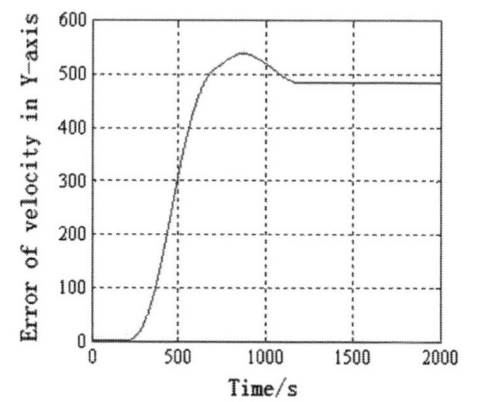

Fig. 5.21 Curve of inertial
navigation z-axis velocity
deviation

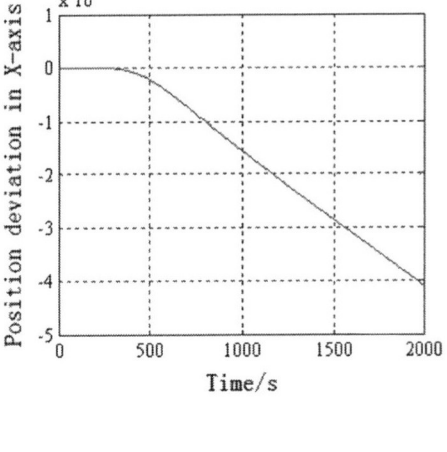

Fig. 5.22 Curve of inertial
navigation x-axis position
error

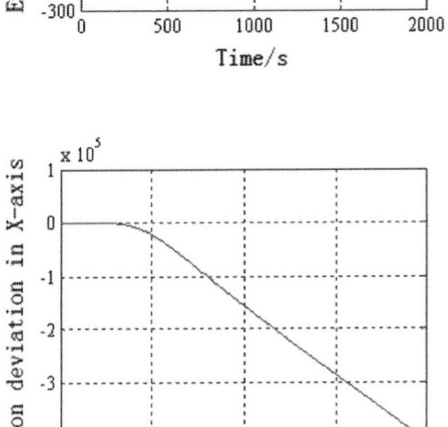

Fig. 5.23 Curve of inertial
navigation y-axis position
error

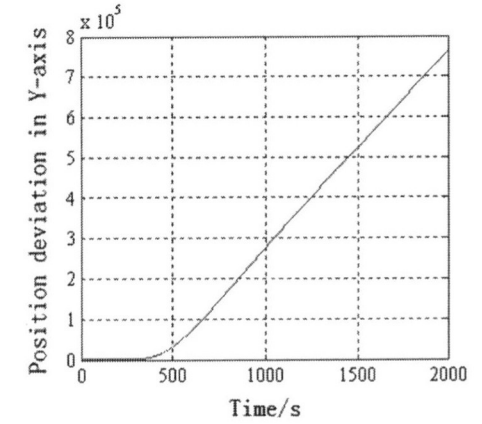

Fig. 5.24 Curve of inertial
z-axis position error

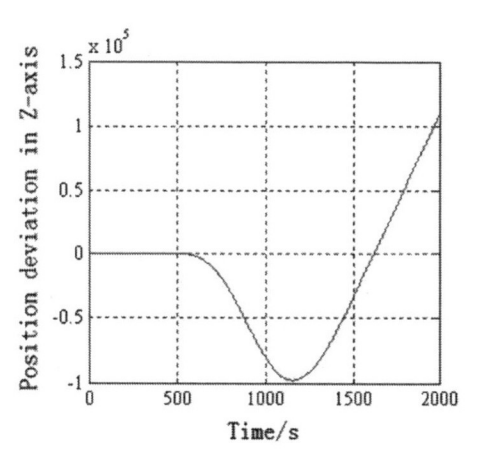

5.5.1   Analysis of Loose Integration Simulation

The mean square deviations of the measurement position and velocity of GPS receiver are 10 m and 0.5 m/s,the measurement cycle is 1 s. When there is no GPS quantity to be measured, only prediction is carried out. The simulation results refer to Figs. 5.25, 5.26, 5.27, 5.28, 5.29, 5.30, 5.31, 5.32 and 5.33.

From the simulation results, we can know that the loose integration could greatly improve the accuracy of navigation of velocity and position. However, because the output correction could not correct the internal error of the INS, the tracking capability of satellite navigation system on the attitude is not high, the correction capability on attitude error is limited.

Fig. 5.25 Deviation curve of
loose integration yaw angle

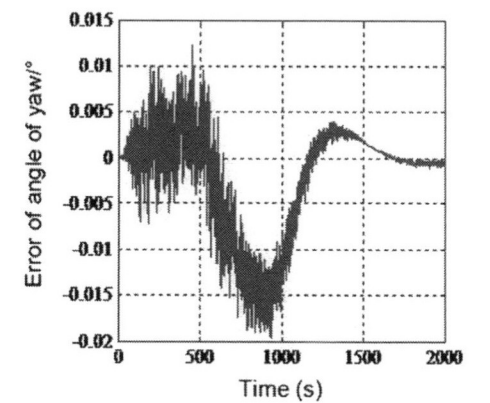

Fig. 5.26 Deviation curve of
loose integration pitch angle

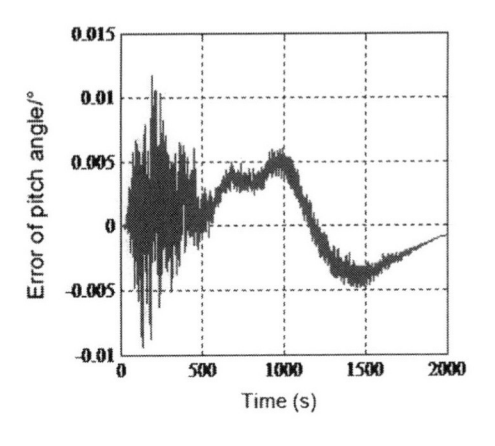

Fig. 5.27 Deviation curve of
loose integration rolling angle

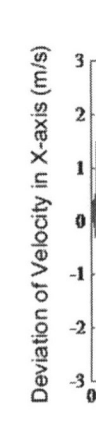

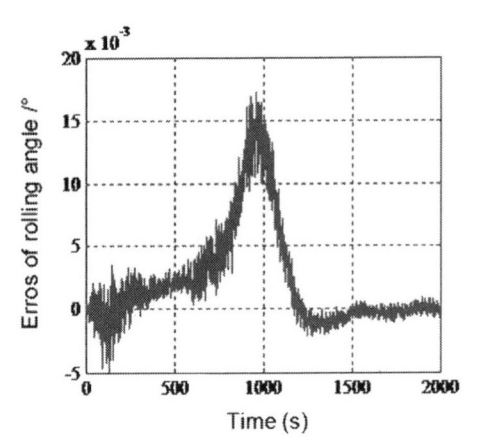

Fig. 5.28 Deviation curve of
loose integration x-axis
velocity

Fig. 5.29 Deviation curve of loose integration y-axis velocity

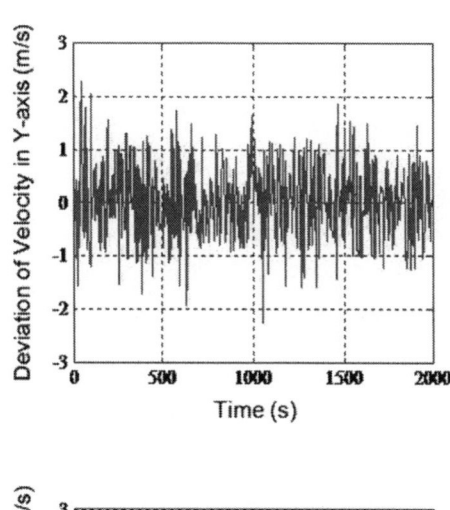

Fig. 5.30 Deviation curve of loose integration z-axis velocity

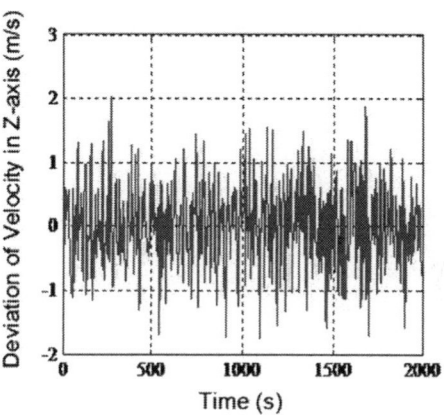

Fig. 5.31 Deviation Curve of Loose Integration x-axis Position

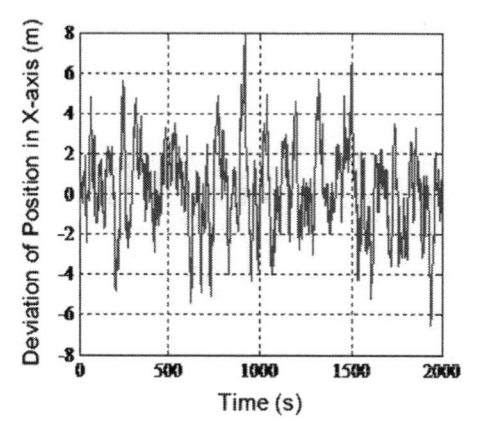

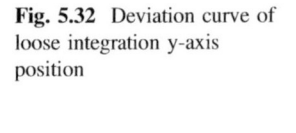

Fig. 5.32 Deviation curve of loose integration y-axis position

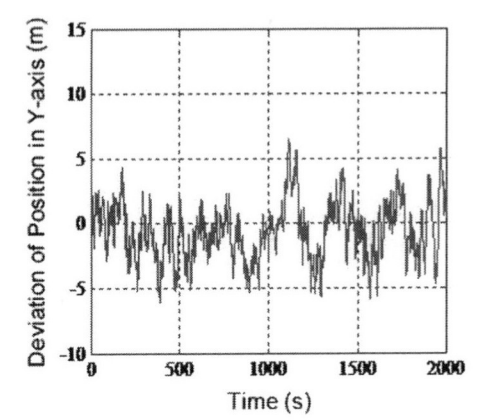

Time (s)

Fig. 5.33 Deviation curve of loose integration z-axis position

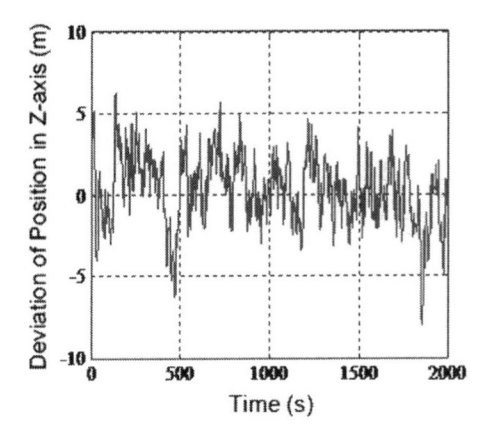

Time (s)

5.5.2 Analysis on Tight Integration Simulation

Take the mean square deviation of measurement pseudo-range and pseudo-range rate of GPS receiver as 10 m and 0.5 m/s, the measurement cycle is 1 s, the initial error of equivalent range of clock offset and distance change range are 5 m and 0.2 m/s respectively, the related time is 50 s. When there is no GSP quantity measured, only prediction is carried out. The simulation results refer to Figs. 5.34, 5.35, 5.36, 5.37, 5.38, 5.39, 5.40, 5.41 and 5.42.

From the simulation results above we can know, compared to pure INS, the tight integration could greatly improve the navigation accuracy of velocity and position. Meanwhile, compared with the mode of loose integration, the difference of navigation effect is not large, and the observation quantity only uses the data of three navigation satellites, which has better anti-interference capability than that of the loose integration mode.

Fig. 5.34 Deviation curve of
tight integration yaw angle

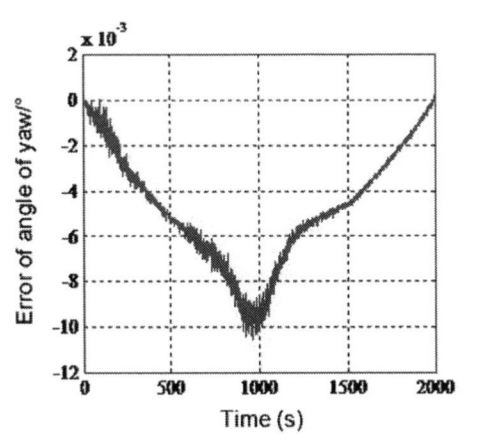

Fig. 5.35 Deviation curve of
tight integration pitch angle

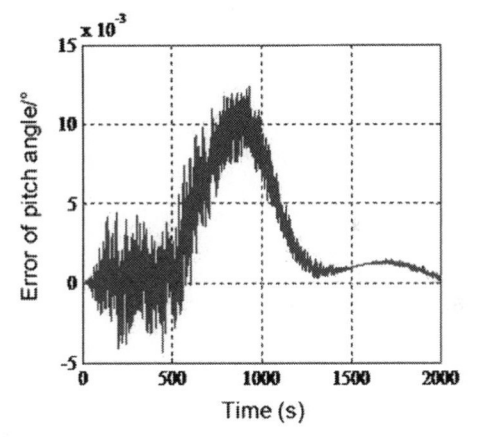

Fig. 5.36 Deviation curve of
tight integration rolling angle

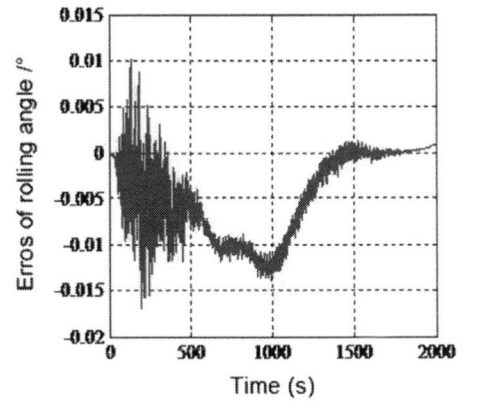

Fig. 5.37 Deviation curve of
tight integration x-axis
velocity

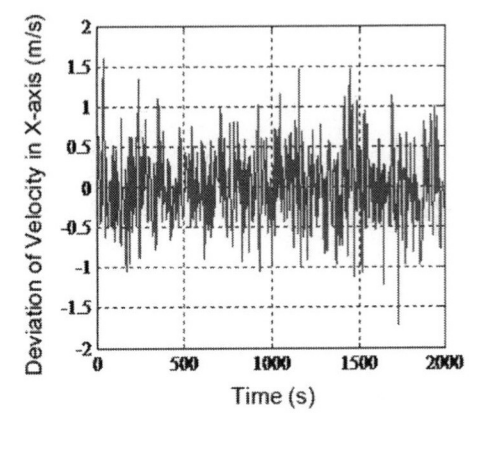

Fig. 5.38 Deviation curve of
tight integration y-axis
velocity

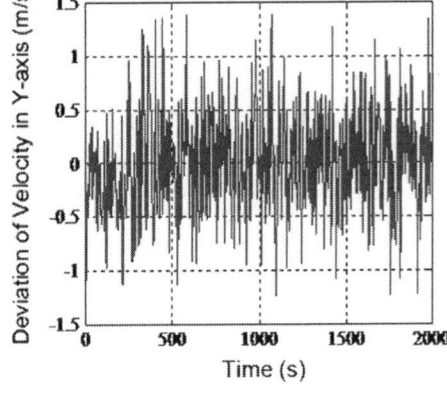

Fig. 5.39 Deviation curve of
tight integration z-axis
velocity

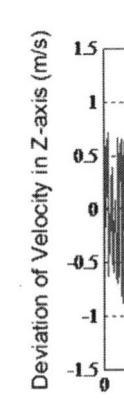
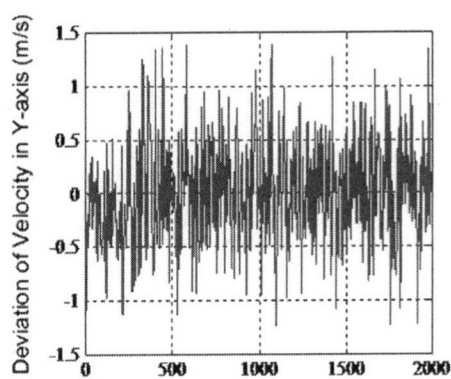

Fig. 5.40 Deviation curve of tight integration x-axis position

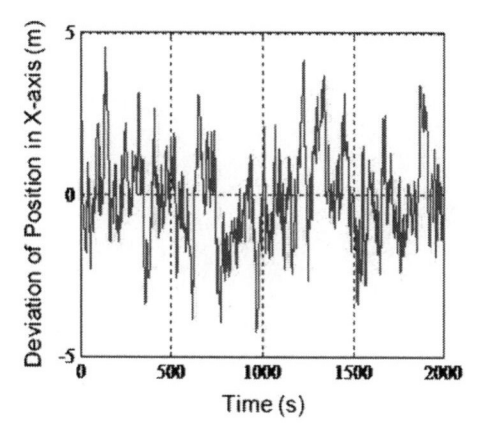

Fig. 5.41 Deviation curve of tight integration y-axis position

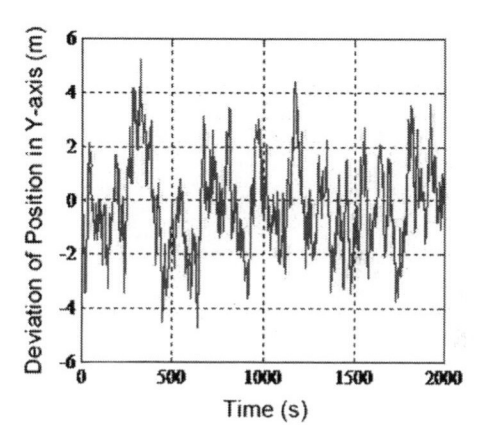

Fig. 5.42 Deviation curve of tight integration z-axis position

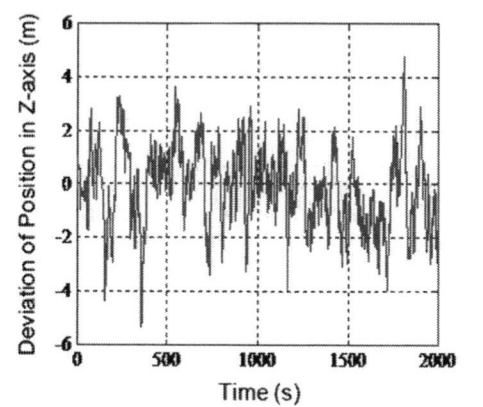

Reference Documentation

1. Quan Wei. 2011. *Inertial, Celestial and Satellite Integrated Navigation Technology*. National Defense Industry Press.
2. Scott Gleason, Demoz Gebre-Egziabher. 2011. *Application and Method of GNSS*. Translated by Yang Dongkai, Fan Jianbin, Zhang Bo, Zhang Min. Electronic Industry Press.
3. Written by Elliott D. Kaplan, Christopher J. Hegarty. 2007. Translated by Kou Yanhong. GPS Principle and Application. Electronic Industry Press.
4. Zhang Qin, Li Jiaquan. 2005. *GPS Measurement Principle and Application*. Science Press.
5. .Chen Shaohua. 2012. *Research on High Orbit Maneuver Vehicle SINS/GPS/CNS Autonomous Navigation Technology*. Nanjing University of Aeronautics and Astronautics.
6. Liao He. 2007. *Research on Algorithm of SINS/GPS Integrated Navigation System of Orbital Transfer Vehicle*. Harbin Institute of Technology.
7. Ma Song. 2010. *Research on SINS/GPS Integrated Navigation System of Space Maneuver Platform*. Harbin Institute of Technology.
8. Gu Zhijun. 2004. *Research on Space-borne Satellite, Inertial Deep Full Integrated Navigation Technology*. National University of Defense Technology.
9. Liu Jianye. 2010. *Theory and Application of Navigation System*. Northwest Industrial University Press.
10. .Zhang Jian. 2009. *Research on Based on GPS Attitude Determination of Flight Vehicle*. Harbin Institute of Technology.

Chapter 6
INS/CNS-Integrated Navigation Technology

6.1 Introduction

When the OTV is at medium high orbit, the navigation satellite signal received by the receiver is relatively weak, even unavailable at certain period. At this moment, the INS/GNSS-integrated navigation technology described in the previous chapter could not be used for improving the accuracy of inertial navigation.

Celestial navigation is the technology of navigation with the celestial information obtained by measuring celestial sensor. Due to the interference factors of atmospheric refraction, which existed in low orbit, celestial navigation is usually used by the flight vehicle in medium and high orbit. Compared with inertial navigation, the error of celestial navigation is not accumulated with time elapses. The integration of INS and CNS is the important means to guarantee the accuracy of navigation system when the satellite navigation signal is unavailable.

This chapter focuses on discussion of starlight navigation technology that relies on star sensor. Based on this, the technology of determining orbit and attitude of orbital transfer vehicle by the integration of inertial navigation, star sensor and auxiliary means are described.

6.2 Starlight Navigation Principle

6.2.1 Starlight Attitude Determination Principle

The star sensor measures the included angle between one reference axis of the fight vehicle and the given star line of sight by sensing the radiation of star. Thus, the star sensor could obtain the azimuth information corresponding to the inertial space. Mount the star sensor on aerospace vehicle, coincide the body axis system with the coordinate system of star sensor; Take the star reference coordinate system as the

© Springer Nature Singapore Pte Ltd. and National Defense Industry Press, Beijing 2018   73
X. Li and C. Li, *Navigation and Guidance of Orbital Transfer Vehicle*, Navigation: Science and Technology, https://doi.org/10.1007/978-981-10-6334-3_6

geocentric inertial coordinate system. The outputs of the star sensor are the three attitude angles of body axis system related to the inertial coordinate system. Commonly, in actual application, the frequently used is the transformation matrix of coordinates of body axis system corresponding to the inertial coordinate system.

The basic process of measurement attitude of star sensor is shown in Fig. 6.1.

First, the optical system images the starlit sky in the field of view on the detector. The later will transform the light signals on each pixel into electrical signals, and coverts into digital via A/D converter, and obtain digital map, which is the result of sampling the image information on the image surface by the detector.

Then, the space-borne computer begins picking up the image, calculating the position and brightness of the image of star observed in star map. The digital map shows the brightness of various pixels with grey level. The brightness of pixel hereby is called gray level in unity. To improve the position accuracy of star image, let the image defocusing, the stellar dispersions are scattered to several pixels. According to

$$x_b = \frac{\sum x_i f(x_i, y_i)}{\sum f(x_i, y_i)}, y_b = \frac{\sum y_i f(x_i, y_i)}{\sum f(x_i, y_i)}$$

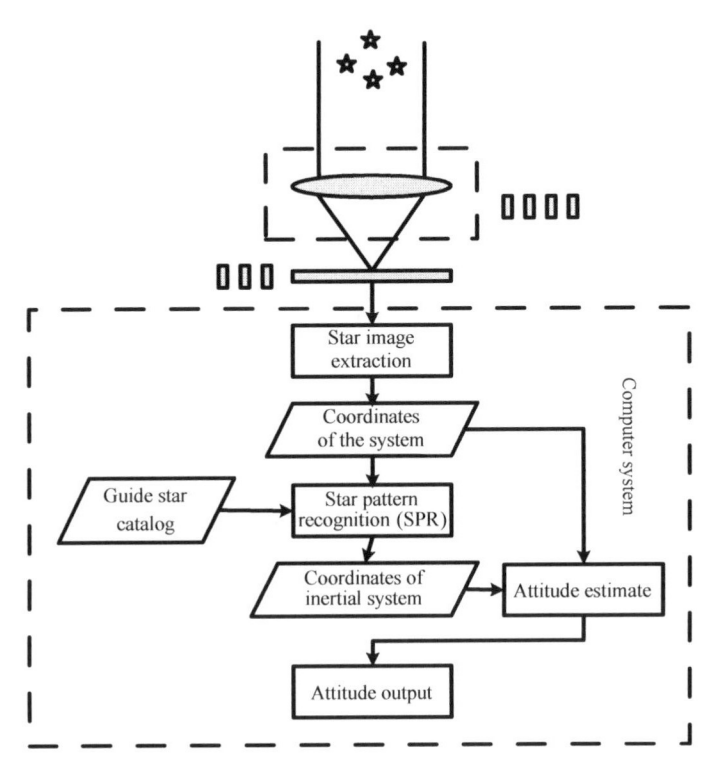

Fig. 6.1 Fundamentals of starlight attitude determination

to solve the luminance centroid of image (x_b, y_b). Among which (x_i, y_i) shows the coordinate of the i pixel of the stellar dispersion of single star on the $X_b Y_b$ plane of the body axis system. $f(x_i, y_i)$ shows the grey level of such pixel.

According to the formula

$$V_b = \begin{bmatrix} V_{bx} \\ V_{by} \\ V_{bz} \end{bmatrix} = \frac{-1}{\sqrt{x_b^2 + y_b^2 + z_b^2}} \begin{bmatrix} x_b \\ y_b \\ -f \end{bmatrix}$$

Obtain the azimuth cosine vector V_b of the observation star in the body axis system. The brightness value of the image is

$$f(x_b, y_b) = \sum f(x_i, y_i)$$

Furthermore, determine the position of observation star in the inertial coordinate system through map identification. At present, multi-observation stars in the field of view form one star team. Based on the azimuth cosine vector V_b of them in the body axis system, the map identification procedure calculates the characteristics of the observation star team, and match with the features of navigation star team. If the matching result is only one, the identification succeeds. The navigation star database keeps the coordinate data of navigation star in the inertial coordinate system. From which, the coordinates of the identified observation star in the inertial coordinate system could be obtained.

Finally, in accordance with the above-mentioned body axis coordinate system of the observation star, the azimuth cosine vector V_b and V_i of the inertial coordinate system, calculate and obtain the rotational relations between the system of proprio-coordinate and the inertial coordinate system, determine the present three axle directions of the star sensor, and complete the attitude estimation.

With the above-mentioned steps, the starlight attitude determined is completed smoothly. The following aspects shall be noticed

1. Establishment and Screening of Guide Star Catalog

Guide Star Catalog is the essential basic data to fulfill CNS navigation functions. Without them, the star map will be incomplete. The star in the Guide Star Catalog is called navigation star. The Guide Star Catalog contains the basic information including the right ascension, declination, and star magnitude of the navigation stars.

The selection of guide stars requires that: (1), the star magnitude shall match with the performance of star sensor, that is, the star observed by the star sensor shall be contained in the Guide Star Catalog. Thus, the star magnitude shall be equal to or higher than the limit stars of the star sensor, etc. Also, the numbers of navigation stars in the field of view could meet the requirement of identification. (2) Under the premise of meeting the normal identification, the star magnitude shall be smaller as possible. Thus, the capacity of Guide Star Catalog could be reduced, and the total

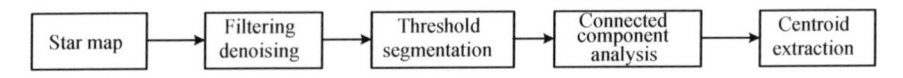

Fig. 6.2 Diagram of star map preprocessing process

number of stars in the Guide Star Catalog could reduce the probability of redundant pairing, further to improve the speed of identification.

2. Star Image Preprocessing

The preprocessing of star image mainly includes noise reduction and star centroid pickup. Since the star map really shot is affected by the factors of dark current of photosensitive devices and celestial background, there exists certain noise, commonly, the noise could be removed by the methods of median filter, linear filter. Then, determine the star coordinates with the centroid extraction algorithm. The entire process is shown in Fig. 6.2.

(1) Filtering Denoising

The star map is shot by CCD camera. The main sources of the star map noise are from the aberration, scattering, diffraction, etc. Noise may deteriorate the quality of image, fuzzy the features of image and bring difficulty for analysis. Thus, before picking up the image features, first of all, carry out filtering. Commonly, carry out filtering after the gray processing of colored star map. Since the gray level of the star in the map is approximately subject to Gaussian distribution. To suppress the noise, the neighborhood average method could be used for filtering denoising.

(2) Threshold Segmentation

To pick up target from star background, one threshold is necessary to separate the star from the image background. If the threshold chosen is too small, redundant information will be collected, while too large threshold will remove some useful information. Thus, one optimum threshold is an important premise of star pickout. Usually, Bemsen algorithm is used to calculate partial threshold. The idea of such algorithm is to find the maximum and the minimum pixel grey levels, and take the average as the threshold of such target pixel.

(3) Connected Component Analysis (CCL)

After obtaining the two values of threshold segmentation, it is necessary to separate the single star from other stars with the Connected Component Analysis (CCA), that is, locate the star target by analyzing the volume and pattern of star, to combine the target pixel contained and separate the target star from other stars. After the CCA, the star targets are the set with the same pixels. To reduce the influence of noise on star extraction, the star whose pixels that are less than or equal to three shall be discarded.

(4) Centroid Extraction

The centroid extraction is the process of obtaining star position by calculating the pixel output signal of the detector. With the star position obtained, the next attitude calculation could be done. Thus, the accuracy of star position extraction directly determines the accuracy of attitude measurement. To obtain higher positioning precision of star, normally, defocus mode is used to scatter the image point of star on CCD light-sensitive surface to more pixels.

3. Star Identification

Star identification is to match the features of the star map formed by stars observed in FOV of the star sensor in real time with that of navigation stars in the database, to determine the relations between observation stars and navigation stars. At present, according to the modes of feature extraction, the methods of star identification is roughly divided into two types, the first is the subgraph isomorphism, that is, take the angular distance between the stars as the edge, and the star as the vertex, the observation star in the field of view is taken as one subgraph of the whole celestial map, which use the information of angular distance directly or indirectly, take the line segments, triangle, or quadrangle as the basic matching elements, and make up the navigation feature database according to certain modes. Such methods mainly include angular polygon algorithm, maximum matching algorithm, triangle algorithm, etc. The second type is the star identification algorithm using star mode. Such algorithm thinks that every star has its own mode, which takes the geometric distribution characteristics of other stars within the domain of the observation star as the characteristic mode of such star. Such method approaches to the model matching problem in a general sense. Among which, the typical one is the grid algorithm.

4. Attitude Determination of Star Sensor

From Fig. 6.1, we can know that, the attitude determination of star sensor needs the information in two aspects, first, the navigation star information in carrier system,

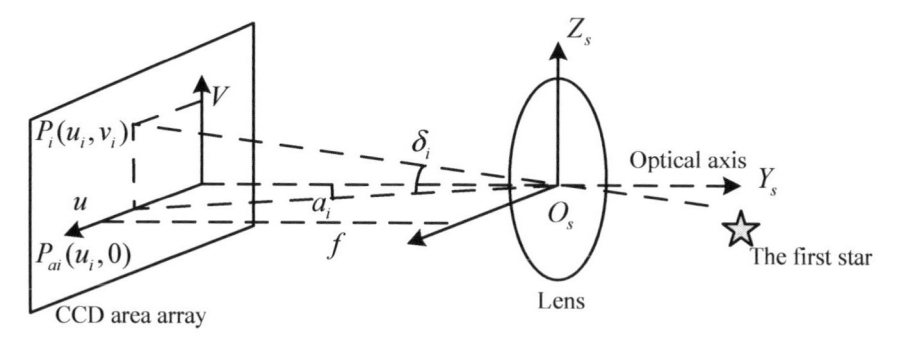

Fig. 6.3 Measurement principle of star sensor

which could be obtained from star sensor. Figure 6.3 shows the measurement mechanism of star sensor.

Extract the image of navigation star on the CCD area array through centroid, and obtain the coordinate of image point (x_c, y_c). Thus, the unit vector of navigation star could be obtained. Such vector is shown in star coordinate system as

$$W_i = \begin{bmatrix} -\sin \alpha_i \cos \delta_i \\ \cos \alpha_i \cos \delta_i \\ -\sin \delta_i \end{bmatrix} = \frac{1}{\sqrt{x_{ci}^2 + y_{ci}^2 + f^2}} \begin{bmatrix} -x_{ci} \\ -y_{ci} \\ f \end{bmatrix} \tag{6.2.1}$$

Here, W_i is called observation vector. Here, f is the focus of star-sensitive optical lens, the definitions of α and δ are shown in the Figure. They are the two angles formed by star vector with the coordinate axle and coordinate plane during the process of star observation.

After obtaining the navigation star information in carrier system, the attitude determination calculation also needs the navigation star information in inertial system. Through star identification, coordinate (GHA, δ) of the target image corresponding to the star in celestial coordinate system. GHA and δ are the Greenwich hour angle and declination of such star in inertial system at the moment of shooting. The position coordinate of the star unit vector in geocentric inertial system is shown as

$$V_i = \begin{bmatrix} \cos GHA_i \cos \delta_i \\ \sin GHA_i \cos \delta_i \\ \sin \delta_i \end{bmatrix} \tag{6.2.2}$$

Here, V_i is called reference vector.

If given the positions of two or multi-stars, we could determine the attitude transformation matrix from inertial coordinate system to star sensor coordinate system, and further solve the inertial attitude of the flight vehicle, i.e., the output attitude angle of star sensor. In solving the attitude of the OTV, one common issue frequently met is how to solve the transformation matrix of coordinates from the measurement of a series of vectors. Such transformation matrix of coordinates shall meet the Eq. (6.2.3),

$$AV_i = W_i, \quad i = 1, \cdots, n \tag{6.2.3}$$

From the above-mentioned analysis, we can easily see that, $W_1, \cdots, W_n$ and $V_1, \cdots, V_n$ show the coordinates measured of the same n vectors in star coordinate system (coinciding with the body axis system) and reference coordinate system (commonly the inertial system). The solving process of Matrix A, that is to solve the transformation matrix of coordinate from body axis system to inertial system. The common methods for attitude solution are the TRAID Algorithm, Multi-vector Attitude Determination Algorithm, q Method, QUEST Directional Vector, etc.

6.2.2   Principle of Starlight Positioning

The star sensor could only directly measure the attitude information. As for the OTV, horizontal direction is very important observation quantity. By sensing the horizon, we could obtain the information of OTV position.

The modes of sensing horizon commonly consist of direct sensing horizon and indirect sensing horizon.

Direct sensing horizon is commonly referred to obtain the direction of geocentric vector in flight vehicle body coordinate by applying infrared earth sensor for measuring the tangential direction of vehicle vertical direction or the edge of vehicle to the edge of the Earth. According to the geometric relations among the flight vehicle, observed navigation star and the ear, in combination with the orbital dynamic equation and filter estimation method, we could obtain the high precise navigation information of velocity, position, etc.

Commonly, indirect sensing horizon refers to applying starlight refraction that is when the starlight crosses the atmosphere of the Earth, due to the uneven density of the atmosphere, the star light observed on the flight vehicle will have refraction, bending to the geocentric direction, which shifts the apparent position of star up than the actual position. If the refraction angle of one known star that is close to horizontal direction is obtained, we could calculate the apparent altitude of the refracted light corresponding to that of the Earth. Such apparent altitude is just the function of the position of the flight vehicle. Through a series of observation data and in combination with the filtering by orbital dynamic equation, the navigation information of the vehicle position, velocity could be obtained.

1. Principle of Direct Sensing Horizon

As shown in Fig. 6.4, in the commonly used direct sensing horizon method, the starlight angle β (the included angle between star visual line and the direction of geocentric vector) is taken as the observation quantity. From the geometric relation, the specific expression is

$$\beta = \arccos\left(-\frac{\mathbf{r} \bullet \mathbf{s}}{r}\right) \tag{6.2.4}$$

Here $\mathbf{r}$ is the position vector of flight vehicle in geocentric inertial coordinate system, which is measured by earth sensor. $\mathbf{s}$ is the unit vector of the starlight direction of navigation star, which is measured by star sensor.

2. Principle of Indirect Sensing Horizon

When starlight crosses the atmosphere of the earth, the light will deviate toward geocentric direction. Seen from the orbit, when the real position of star goes down, its apparent position remains above the horizon. The apparent altitude of the refracted light observed from the flight vehicle corresponding to the earth is h_a, actually, it is at one lower height h_g from the ground, as shown in Fig. 6.5.

Fig. 6.4 Observation model
of direct sensing horizon

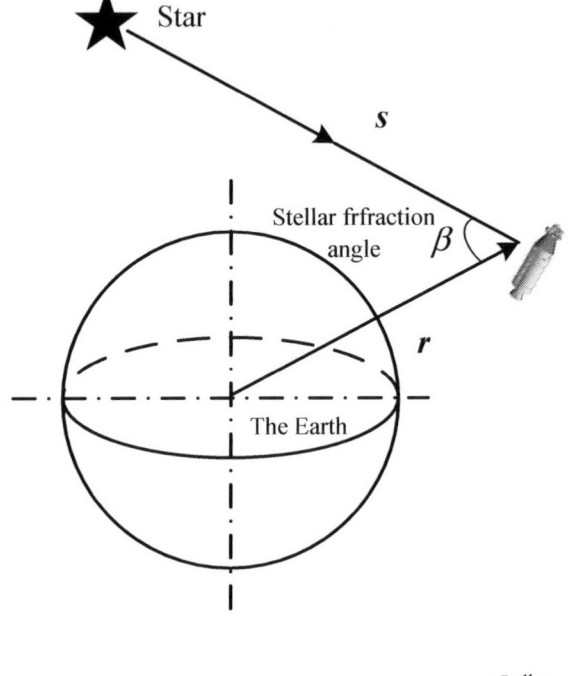

Fig. 6.5 Starlight refraction
geometric relations

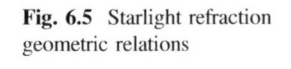

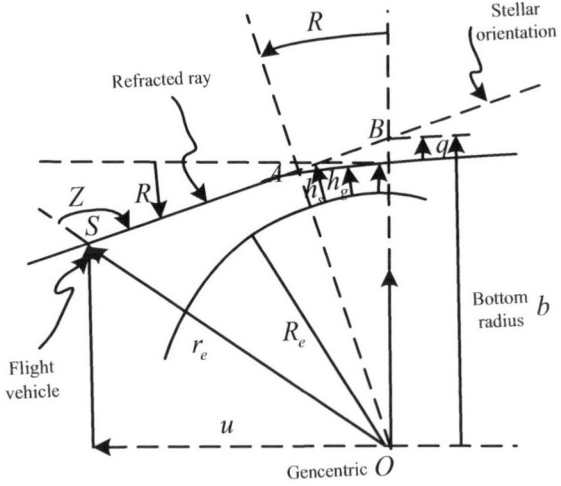

The purpose of measuring starlight refraction angle is that it has contained the information related to position of flight vehicle, while there is no direction geometric relations between the refraction angle R and starlight refraction height h_g with the position of flight vehicle, only could the apparent height h_a play the role of bridge that connects the refraction angle R and the position of flight vehicle. Specifically, it has

$$h_a(R, \rho) = h_0 - H \ln(R) + H \ln[k(\lambda)\rho_0(\frac{2\pi R_e}{H})^{\frac{1}{2}}] + R(\frac{HR_e}{2\pi})^{\frac{1}{2}} \tag{6.2.5}$$

Here ρ_0 is the density of height h_0, H is the scale height of density, $k(\lambda)$ is the scattering parameter. The above-mentioned formula reveals the relations between apparent height h_a, refraction angle R, and atmosphere density ρ.

In addition, from Fig. 6.5 we can see

$$h_a = \sqrt{r_s^2 - u^2} + u \tan(R) - R_e - a \tag{6.2.6}$$

Here $u = |r_s \cdot u_s|$, r_s is the position vector of flight vehicle, and u_s is the direction vector of the starlight before refraction.

Equations (6.2.5) and (6.2.6) established the relations of measuring refraction quantity and the vehicle position, which is essential to apply the starlight refraction for positioning of the OTV.

While applying the starlight refraction for navigation of flight vehicle, not only one set of complete star map is needed, but also it needs to establish the atmosphere refraction model. The final navigation precision is determined by the measurement error, the quantity of refracted starlight and direction, and the types of orbits of flight vehicle, etc.

6.3   Design of INS/CNS-Integrated Navigation System

The observation quantity of star sensor could accurately obtain the attitude relations between the body axis system and inertial frame of reference, so as to correct the gyroscope drift of the inertial frame of reference, to improve the attitude accuracy of the navigation system. Although the factors of aberration, procession, and nutation of the Earth polar axis have tiny change of the star direction, the attitude error caused is less than $1''$. Therefore, substantially, the star sensor equals to the gyroscope without drift, which could be used for correcting the attitude error of the INS. The common mode is to take the error of attitude information obtained by SINS and star sensor as the measurement, via estimation of filter and make compensation for the attitude error of SINS and gyroscope drift.

The INS and star sensor of the OTV are usually installed in the mode of strapdown, that is, to adopt the full strapdown work mode. At this moment, from the attitude information transmitted by star sensor, we could obtain the information of attitude of the three axles of the flight vehicle (pitch angle φ, course angle ψ and roll angle γ). Subtract the two and obtain the attitude error angle $\Delta\varepsilon$ of the three axles of the carrier

$$\Delta \varepsilon = \begin{bmatrix} \varepsilon_\varphi \\ \varepsilon_\psi \\ \varepsilon_\gamma \end{bmatrix} = \begin{bmatrix} \varphi - \varphi_0 \\ \psi - \psi_0 \\ \gamma - \gamma_0 \end{bmatrix} \tag{6.3.1}$$

Since the error model of strapdown inertial navigation system is the misalignment angle of mathematical platform, the attitude error angle could be taken as the observation quantity of integrated navigation filter by converted into misalignment angle of mathematical platform, the expression of attitude error angle transforming into mathematical platform misalignment angle is

$$\varphi = \begin{bmatrix} \varphi_x \, \varphi_y \, \varphi_z \end{bmatrix}^{\mathrm{T}} = M \bullet \Delta \varepsilon \tag{6.3.2}$$

Here M is the transformation matrix of attitude error angle

$$M = \begin{bmatrix} 0 & \cos \varphi & -\cos \psi \sin \varphi \\ 0 & \sin \varphi & \cos \psi \cos \varphi \\ 1 & 0 & \sin \psi \end{bmatrix}$$

The schematic diagram of INS/CNS-integrated navigation is shown in Fig. 6.6. In such integrated mode, the SINS error equation is taken as the integrated system state equation, the mathematical platform misalignment angle is the measurement value of the system. Commonly, the output frequency of the star sensor is lower than that of the original data including acquisition angle increment, apparent velocity of the INS, usually, after the SINS subsystem calculates several cycles, input the results calculated with the data of star sensor into the optimal estimation filter. Through the estimation of the filter, correct the mathematical platform misalignment angle of the SINS, meanwhile, estimate the drift error of the three gyroscopes. Then, correct the measurement information of the gyroscope directly.

Takes the launching inertial system as the navigation coordinate system, the state equation of the integrated navigation system is the same as that in Sect. 5.4.1. The observation quantity is the attitude misalignment angle φ, the observation equation of the attitude is

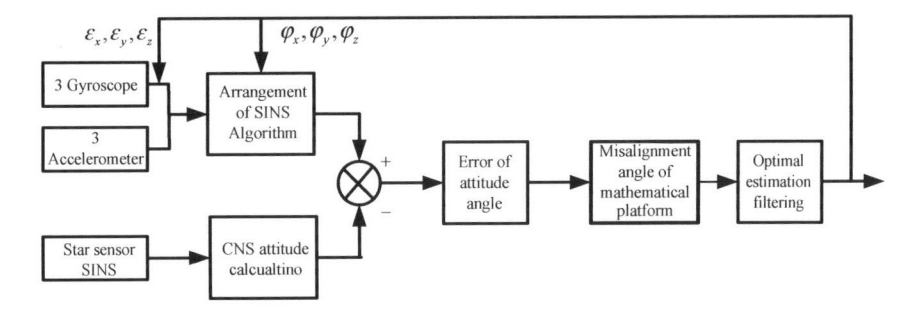

Fig. 6.6 Schematic diagram of INS/CNS-integrated navigation

$$Z_a(t) = \left[\varphi_x \; \varphi_y \; \varphi_z\right]^{\mathrm{T}} = H_a X(t) + V_a(t) \tag{6.3.3}$$

Here $H_a = [I_{3\times3} \quad 0_{3\times12}]$, V_a is the measurement noise of star sensor. After estimating the misalignment angle and gyroscope drift according to the state and observation equations, the next step is to correct the output of the mathematical platform and gyroscope.

1. Correction of Mathematical Platform

Since the misalignment angle is usually small, assumes the attitude matrix before and after the correction are the respective $C_b^{n_1}$ and $C_b^{n_2}$, from the error analysis of the SINS in Sect. 4.2.3, there is

$$C_b^{n_2} = \begin{bmatrix} 1 & -\varphi_z & \varphi_y \\ \varphi_z & 1 & -\varphi_x \\ -\varphi_y & \varphi_x & 1 \end{bmatrix} C_b^{n_1} \tag{6.3.4}$$

Use Eq. (6.3.4), we could correct the strapdown attitude matrix.

The estimation of SINS mathematical platform misalignment angle may use quaternion error compensation method. The quaternion before compensation is q_1, from the rotational quaternion theorem we could know the quaternion compensated is

$$q_2 = q_1 \left(1 + \frac{\varphi_x}{2}\bar{i} + \frac{\varphi_y}{2}\bar{j} + \frac{\varphi_z}{2}\bar{k}\right) \tag{6.3.5}$$

Being expanded, obtain

$$\begin{cases} q_{20} = q_{10} - q_{11}\dfrac{\varphi_x}{2} - q_{12}\dfrac{\varphi_y}{2} - q_{13}\dfrac{\varphi_z}{2} \\[2mm] q_{21} = -q_{10}\dfrac{\varphi_x}{2} + q_{11} - q_{12}\dfrac{\varphi_z}{2} - q_{13}\dfrac{\varphi_y}{2} \\[2mm] q_{22} = q_{10}\dfrac{\varphi_y}{2} + q_{11}\dfrac{\varphi_z}{2} + q_{12} - q_{13}\dfrac{\varphi_x}{2} \\[2mm] q_{23} = q_{10}\dfrac{\varphi_z}{2} - q_{11}\dfrac{\varphi_y}{2} + q_{12}\dfrac{\varphi_x}{2} + q_{13} \end{cases} \tag{6.3.6}$$

Then, through normalization processing, obtain

$$\hat{q}_2 = \frac{q_2}{|q_2|} \tag{6.3.7}$$

Equations (6.3.6) and (6.3.7) form the process of correcting the attitude error angle. $\hat{q}_2$ is the corrected quaternion.

2. Correction of Gyroscope Output

The output quantity of gyroscope before and after the correction are $\omega_x, \omega_y, \omega_z$ and $\hat{\omega}_x, \hat{\omega}_y, \hat{\omega}_z$ respectively, then,

$$\begin{cases} \hat{\omega}_x = \omega_x - \varepsilon_x \\ \hat{\omega}_y = \omega_y - \varepsilon_y \\ \hat{\omega}_z = \omega_z - \varepsilon_z \end{cases} \tag{6.3.8}$$

After obtaining the corrected state quantity, continue the next navigation calculation.

6.4 Analysis of Simulation Results

First, design the trajectory of the flight vehicle and take navigation coordinate system as the launching inertial system. Assumes the longitude of the launch point of flight vehicle is 118°, latitude is 32°, the initial height is 0 m and launching azimuth is 90°. Simulate one flight section of the flight vehicle and the simulation time is 600 s. In terms of the established trajectory, take the constant drift of gyroscope as 0.2°/h, the mean square root of white noise is 0.2°/h; the error of starlight error meter 21″. The calculating period of inertial navigation is 0.02 s. The simulated trajectory and simulation results are shown in Figs. 6.7, 6.8, 6.9, 6.10, 6.11, 6.12, and 6.13.

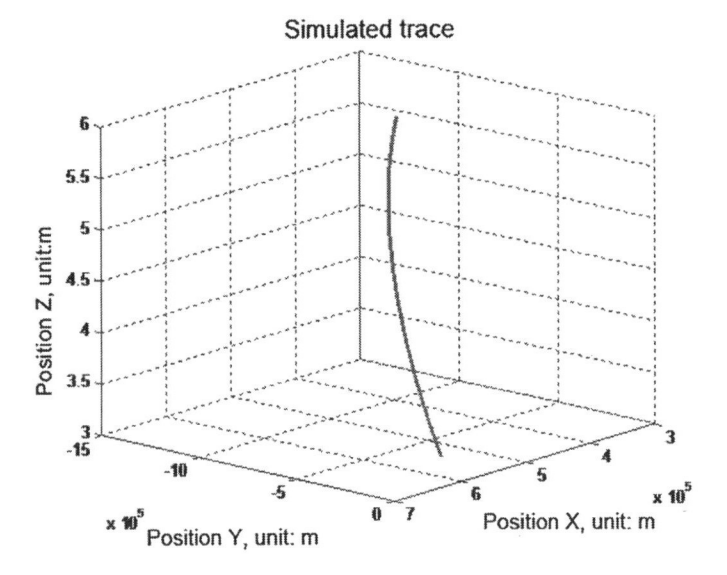

Fig. 6.7 Simulated trace

Fig. 6.8 Error of inertial yaw angle

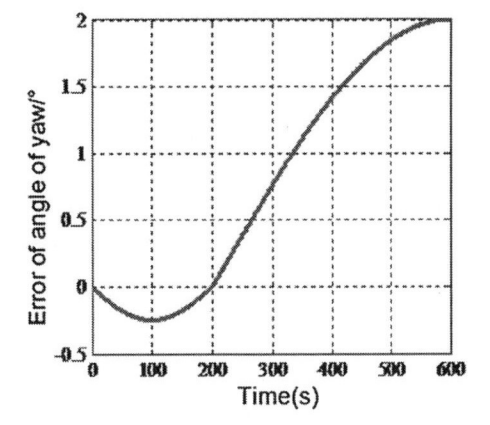

Fig. 6.9 Error of inertial pitch angle

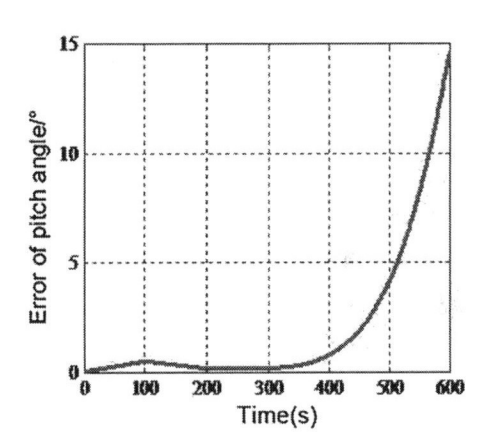

Fig. 6.10 Error of inertial rolling angle

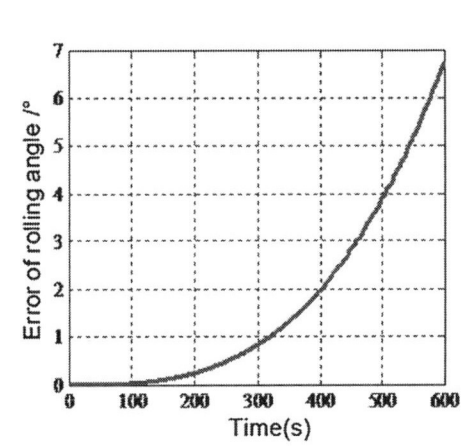

Fig. 6.11 Error of integrated navigation yaw angle

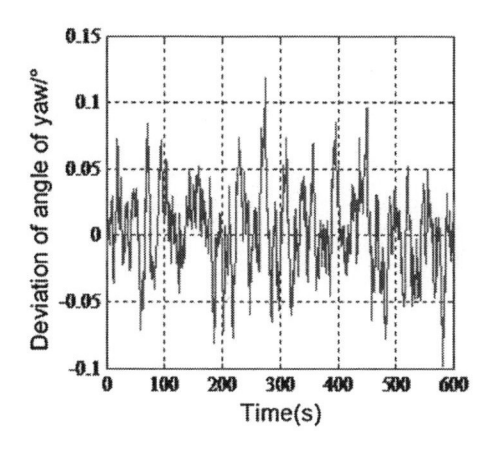

Fig. 6.12 Error of integrated navigation pitch angle

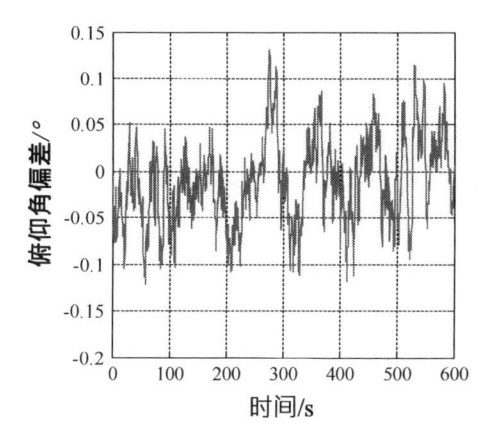

Fig. 6.13 Error of integrated navigation rolling angle

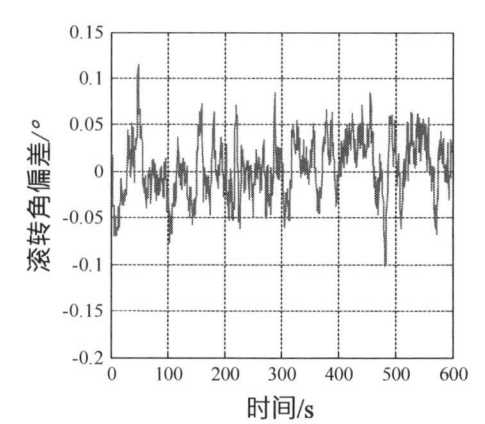

From the above-mentioned simulation results we can know, compared with pure INS, the INS/CNS-integrated navigation system could greatly improve the navigation accuracy, correct the instrumental error effectively, and could fulfill the navigation missions with higher requirement.

Reference Documentation

1. Li Yijie. 2012. Research on Autonomous Navigation Filtering Algorithm of Large Elliptical Orbit Vehicle. Harbin Institute of Technology.
2. Zhang Cheng. 2012. Research on INS/CNS Integrated Navigation Technology of Aerospace Vehicle. Nanjing University of Aeronautics and Astronautics.
3. Fang Jiancheng, Ning Xiaolin. 2006. *Celestial Navigation Principle and Applications*. Beihang University Press.
4. Zhang Libin. 2010. Rocket Upper-stage Navigation, Research on Midcourse Correction and Attitude Control. Harbin Institute of Technology.
5. Qian Yingjing. 2013. Research on Autonomous Navigation and Station keeping For Quasi-periodic Orbit in The Earth-Moon System. Harbin Institute of Technology.
6. Chen Shaohau. 2012. Research on SINS/GPS/CNS Autonomous Navigation Technology of High-orbital Maneuver Vehicle. Nanjing University of Aeronautics and Astronautics.
7. Zhou Baolin. 2009. Research on Semi-physical Situation of INS/CNS Integrated Navigation System. Harbin Institute of Technology.
8. Xueyuan, Jian, Ma. Guangfu, and Luo Jing. 2003. Model of Attitude Measurement Error of Infrared Horizon Sensor. *Journal of Aerospace* 24 (2): 138–143.
9. Tang Qiong. 2007. Determination of Vehicle Autonomous Orbit Based on Starlight Refraction. Northwestern Polytechnical University.

Chapter 7
Redundant Fault Tolerance and Failure Reconfiguration Technology of Inertial Devices

7.1 Introduction

As precision instrument and equipment, the Inertial Navigation System (INS) not only has high accuracy index, but also possess high working reliability. Commonly, there are two methods to improve reliability of the INS, one is to increase the reliability of single device and reduce the rate of occurrence of failures (ROCOF). The second is to adopt the concept of tolerance design, by adding additional hardware resources and algorithm in the system. In case one component in the system fails, the system test and reconfigure the fault through redundant components and algorithms, and reach the purpose of absorbing or isolating fault. Restricted by manufacturing technology, there is limited space to guarantee the reliability of INS by improving reliability of single component. Many studies show that redundant technique has apparent effects for improving the reliability of system.

The redundant scheme of inertial device mainly contains three aspects, one is the redundant configuration, which needs to determine the quantity of redundant devices and its mode of installation. The second is the fault diagnosis. Once fault occurs, the system needs to test and locate the faulty information. The third is the fault reconfiguration. After detecting the fault, it needs to reconfigure the redundant inertial devices to provide the information of correct measurement.

According to the redundant configuration, the redundant scheme of the INS could be divided into single-table redundancy and system-level redundancy. The Strapdown Inertial Navigation System (SINS) adopts the single-table redundant design, which have redundant configuration for single inertial component in Strapdown Inertial Measurement Unit (SIMU) including gyroscope and accelerometer. It could be realized that when certain component fails, the INS could still output the information of angular velocity and acceleration of the carrier normally. The system-level redundancy refers to the redundant system formed by

© Springer Nature Singapore Pte Ltd. and National Defense Industry Press, Beijing 2018
X. Li and C. Li, *Navigation and Guidance of Orbital Transfer Vehicle*, Navigation:
Science and Technology, https://doi.org/10.1007/978-981-10-6334-3_7

multi-SIMUs. When certain SIMU fails, other SIMUs may output the information of angular velocity and acceleration as well.

This chapter lays stress on discussing the management plans of multi-level redundancy of single SIMU and system-level redundancy of multi-sets of SIMUs.

7.2 Redundant Configuration of Inertial Devices

Redundant configuration of inertial devices is to study how to configure the numbers and modes of installation of redundant devices. In case one or multiple inertial devices break down, the system could obtain sufficient measurement information from other inertial devices that work normally. Processing with the mathematical method, the output of acceleration and angular velocity in all the three orthogonal directions is obtained. The starting point of configuration is that, no matter normal or not, the system shall have sufficient information sources of measurement, to guarantee the measurement information used by navigation, and the navigation error and performance are within the range of the allowable precision. With regards to the demands of engineering practice, the process of configuration shall give consideration to economy, complexity, and realizability, that is, under the premise that the information of measurement could be reconfigured and the reconfigured information meet certain accuracy, the number of redundant devices configured shall be minimized and the mode of installation shall be as simple as possible.

As for the INS in aerospace, the common configuration of inertial devices is to install gyroscope and accelerometer, respectively, along the three orthogonal reference axles, to measure the angular velocity along the X-axis, Y-axis, and Z-axis and the acceleration along three directions of X, Y, and Z which is shown Fig. 7.1. We can know that in case one axial gyroscope (accelerometer) fails, the other two

Fig. 7.1 Configuration of common INS

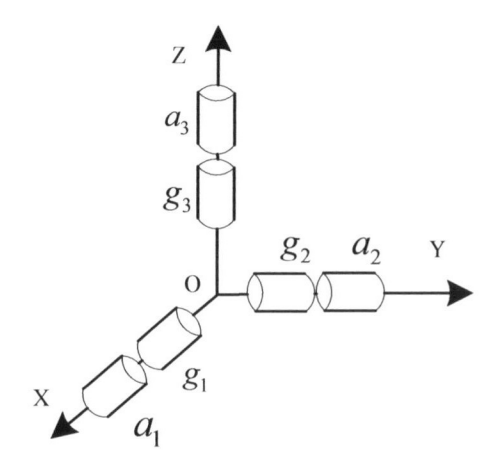

Fig. 7.2 a System-level redundant configuration. **b** Single-table redundant configuration

axial gyroscopes (accelerometers) could not obtain the angular velocity quantity (acceleration) of such direction, by then, the INS will not work normally.

One intuitive redundant configuration method is to increase N inertial devices for each direction, and form N sets of the identical INSs, which is shown in Fig. 7.2a. As mentioned above, this is the system-level redundant configuration. Another idea is to increase the several skewed measurement axle on the basis of the three orthogonal axle, refers to Fig. 7.2b. When the inertial device on the orthogonal axis fails, measure the projection on the orthogonal axis with the device on inclined axis, the state output of such direction could be obtained as well, this is the multi-table redundant configuration.

7.2.1 Multi-table Redundant Configuration of Single Inertial Group

The multi-table redundant configuration of single inertial group mainly consists of two aspects, one is the configuration of instrument number, and the other is the configuration of mounting geometry of instrument. Studies have shown that under the condition of the same reliability index of single device, the volume, weight, and cost of the INS will increase along with the increase in the number of inertial devices. Therefore, in selecting the redundant system, it needs to choose the number of redundant single-table inertial devices. In addition, when the numbers of inertial sensors are the same while the mounting geometry is different, the accuracy of measurement and navigation performance will also be different.

1. Common Configurations

(1) Cone Structure

When the number of sensors is more than 4 (usually 5 or 6), mount the sensors in element of cone on conical surface with one cone angle α along its measurement axis which is shown in Fig. 7.3.

(2) Regular Dodecahedron Structure of Six Sensors

Put the measurement axle of the 6 sensors perpendicular to the parallel plane of the Regular Dodecahedron mutually, which is shown in Fig. 7.4.

(3) Three Orthogonal Multi-inclined Scheme

The six sensors are on the directions of three mutually orthogonal X-, Y-, Z-coordinate axles. Other sensors shall keep certain included angle with the three axles which is shown in Fig. 7.5.

Fig. 7.3 Five-gyroscope cone mounting structural diagram

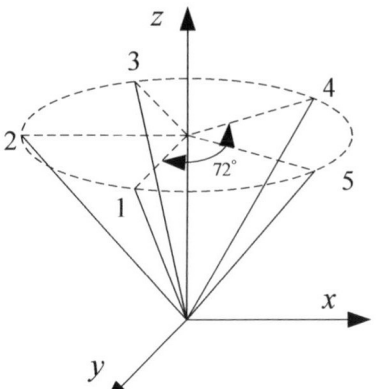

Fig. 7.4 Regular dodecahedron mounting plan

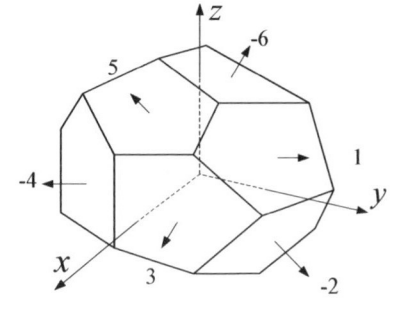

Fig. 7.5 Three-orthogonal
multi-inclined structural
mounting diagram

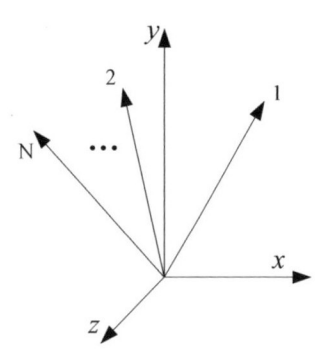

2. Navigation Performance Index

To obtain the optimal navigation performance, first, we should define the measurement equation of the system. It is assumed that the redundant measurement equation formed by m inertial devices is with the same accuracy. Its measurement equation contains noise interference, that is,

$$Z = H\omega + \varepsilon \qquad (7.2.1)$$

In it, $\omega \in R^n$ is the system state to be measured; $Z \in R^m$ is the measurement value of m inertial devices $(m > n)$; $H \in R^{m \times n}$ is the mounting matrix of device configuration, that is the column full rank matrix; ε is the Gaussian white noise sequence zero of m-dimension mean value, covariance $\sigma^2 I_m$, i.e., $E(\varepsilon) = 0, E(\varepsilon \varepsilon^T) = \sigma^2 I_m, I_m$ is the m identity matrix.

If the optimized configuration mounting matrix H minimizes the navigation error of the system aroused by noise, the system will have the optimum navigation performance. Under the situation of no fault, the navigation errors aroused by noise mainly have following three types of performance index:

(1) Assuming the measurement noise as $\varepsilon = (e_1, e_2, \cdots, e_m)^T$, various components are the random constant that are mutually independent, its performance indices are

$$F_{P1} = \sqrt{E_x^2 + E_y^2 + E_z^2} = \sqrt{\sum_{i=1}^{3} \sum_{j=1}^{m} M_{ij}^2} \qquad (7.2.2)$$

Here $\qquad M = (H^T H)^{-1} H^T, E_x = \sqrt{\sum_{j=1}^{m} M_{1j}^2 e_j^2}, E_y = \sqrt{\sum_{j=1}^{m} M_{2j}^2 e_j^2}, E_z = \sqrt{\sum_{j=1}^{m} M_{3j}^2 e_j^2}$, H is the mounting matrix. To measure the effects of noise on three coordinate axles, based on this, extend to include the performance index with weighted factor.

$$F_{P1}^* = \sqrt{a_1 E_x^2 + a_2 E_y^2 + a_3 E_z^2} \tag{7.2.3}$$

(2) Assuming ε is the random vector with mean zero, variance σ^2, performance index is

$$F_{P2} = \sum_{i=1}^{3} a_i G(i, i) \tag{7.2.4}$$

Here a_i is the weighted factor, $G^{-1} = H^T H$, $G(i, i)$ is the i diagonal entry of G.

(3) Given the accuracy of inertial element, the influence of measurement error on orthogonal axle directly relies on the volume of $(H^T H)^{-1}$. The common one is the Gaussian random vector that assumed ε is the mean zero. Define the following performance index

$$F_{P3} = \sqrt{|G|} \tag{7.2.5}$$

Under certain conditions, the above-mentioned three types of navigation error are equivalent. To unify the standard, such period adopts the performance index F_{P1} for the optimized design. That is to choose

$$F_{P1} = \sqrt{E_x^2 + E_y^2 + E_z^2} = \sqrt{\sum_{i=1}^{3} \sum_{j=1}^{m} M_{ij}^2} \tag{7.2.6}$$

When one group of measurement assembly in the system breaks down, such indicator function is applicable, which needs to be improved. Thus, when one group of measurement assembly fails, its performance index is

$$F_p(m, 1) = \sqrt{\frac{1}{m} \left(\sum_{n=1}^{m} E_T^2(n) \right)} \tag{7.2.7}$$

In it, $E_T^2(n) = \sqrt{\sum_{i=1}^{3} \sum_{j=1}^{m} M_{nij}^2}$.

F_P shows the mean square norm of noise measured. Thus, smaller the F_{P1} the lesser the navigation error, the better navigation performance is. Under the situation of orthogonal-inclined configuration, the optimized design is how to select the relations of relative positions between gyroscope sensing axis and orthogonal axis, so as to minimize the measurement error F_P of the redundant system and optimize the performance index of navigation.

3. Optimal Conditions of Navigation Performance Index

Following proves that when $H^TH = \frac{n}{3}I_{3\times3}$, the navigation performance index is the optimal, n is the total number of redundant devices.

Since,

(1) Sufficiency: Let us assume $H^TH = \frac{n}{3}I_{3\times3}$ and the characteristic value of H^TH is $\lambda_1, \lambda_2, \lambda_3$. From the relation

$$\frac{(x+y+z)}{3} \geq \sqrt[3]{xyz} \tag{7.2.8}$$

Obtain the equation

$$J = \text{trace}(P) = \sigma^2 \text{trace}\left\{\left(HH^T\right)^{-1}\right\} = \sigma^2\left(\frac{1}{\lambda_1} + \frac{1}{\lambda_2} + \frac{1}{\lambda_3}\right) \geq \frac{3\sigma^2}{\sqrt[3]{\lambda_1\lambda_2\lambda_3}} \tag{7.2.9}$$

When $\lambda_1 = \lambda_2 = \lambda_3$ equality is established. Thus, when $\lambda_1 = \lambda_2 = \lambda_3 = \frac{n}{3}$, the performance index of navigation J takes the minimal value. Such matrix H is the optimal measurement matrix of navigation performance index.

(2) Necessity: Given $\text{trace}(HH^T) = trace(H^TH) = \sum_{i=1}^{n}\|h_i\|^2 = n$, and

$$\text{trace}\left(HH^T\right) = \lambda_1 + \lambda_2 + \lambda_3 \tag{7.2.10}$$

From $\lambda_1 = \lambda_2 = \lambda_3$ and $\lambda_1 + \lambda_2 + \lambda_3 = n$, obtain $\lambda_1 = \lambda_2 = \lambda_3 = \frac{n}{3}$. To prove that $H^TH = \frac{n}{3}I_{3\times3}$ is established. From decomposing singular values, the measurement matrix could be decomposed as $H = UAV^T$, Here, $U = [u_1, u_2, \ldots u_n]$, $V = [v_1, v_2, \ldots v_n]$, $A = \begin{bmatrix} \sum \\ 0 \end{bmatrix}$, and $\sum = \text{diag}\{\rho_1, \rho_2, \rho_3\}$, u_i and the characteristic value at the left and right of the singular value ρ_1 that are related to H. Since matrix H and formula V is the single one, and $\rho_i^2 = \lambda_i$, then,

$$\sum = \text{diag}\left\{\sqrt{\frac{n}{3}}, \sqrt{\frac{n}{3}}, \sqrt{\frac{n}{3}}\right\} \tag{7.2.11}$$

Proves, $H^\mathrm{T}H = VA^\mathrm{T}U^\mathrm{T}UAV^\mathrm{T} = \sum^2 = \frac{n}{3}I_{3\times3}$.

In particular, when $n = 3$, H is the optimal navigation performance index in $I_{3\times3}$ unit matrix, that is, when there are only three mounting axles, the measurement error of orthogonal mounting is the minimum, which conforms to the experience of actual engineering installation.

Following the above, derive the mounting angle of inclined axis with the optimal navigation performance index of three-orthogonal N-inclined mounting plan. X, Y, Z are the three perpendicular orthogonal axes. Within the $OXYZ$ solid space, there are N inclined axes. The included angle between the inclined axes and Y-axis are $\alpha_1, \ldots, \alpha_N$, respectively, and the included angle between the projection and Z-axis in XOZ plane are respectively $\beta_1, \ldots, \beta_N$, refers to Fig. 7.6.

The mounting matrix is

$$H = \begin{bmatrix} 1 & 0 & 0 \\ 0 & 1 & 0 \\ 0 & 0 & 1 \\ \sin\alpha_1\sin\beta_1 & \cos\alpha_1 & \sin\alpha_1\cos\beta_1 \\ \vdots & \vdots & \vdots \\ \sin\alpha_N\sin\beta_N & \cos\alpha_N & \sin\alpha_N\cos\beta_N \end{bmatrix} \tag{7.2.12}$$

Let $H^\mathrm{T}H = \frac{N+3}{3}I_{3\times3}$, obtain following equation set

$$\begin{cases} 1 + \sin^2\alpha_1\sin^2\beta_1 + \cdots + \sin^2\alpha_N\sin^2\beta_N = (N+3)/3 \\ 1 + \cos^2\alpha_1 + \cdots + \cos^2\alpha_N = (N+3)/3 \\ 1 + \sin^2\alpha_1\cos^2\beta_1 + \cdots + \sin^2\alpha_N\cos^2\beta_N = (N+3)/3 \\ \sin\alpha_1\sin\beta_1\cos\alpha_1 + \cdots + \sin\alpha_N\sin\beta_N\cos\alpha_N = 0 \\ \sin^2\alpha_1\sin\beta_1\cos\beta_1 + \cdots + \sin^2\alpha_N\sin\beta_N\cos\beta_N = 0 \\ \sin\alpha_1\cos\alpha_1\cos\beta_1 + \cdots + \sin\alpha_N\cos\alpha_N\cos\beta_N = 0 \end{cases} \tag{7.2.13}$$

Solve the above-mentioned equation set, and obtain the mounting angle of optimal navigation performance. It is necessary to point out that when the number of inclined axle are more, the above equation set are the contradictory equations,

Fig. 7.6 Three-orthogonal multi-inclined structure installation diagram

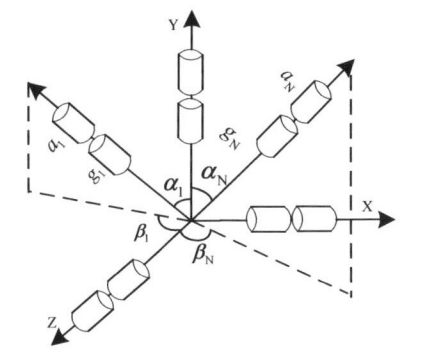

which may have multi groups of different solutions. The specific solution shall be analyzed in particular according to the numbers of inclined axle. When $N = 0$, i.e., there is no redundant inclined mounting axis, the former formula deteriorates to identity, i.e., no redundant configuration is one special case of redundant configuration.

4. Numerical Examples

Taking three orthogonal multi-inclined plan as the example to illustrate the optimal configuration process and related performance index of navigation. When the plan is three-orthogonal one oblique and without fault, commonly β takes $45°$, at this moment, the mounting matrix is

$$
H = \begin{bmatrix}
1 & 0 & 0 \\
0 & 1 & 0 \\
0 & 0 & 1 \\
\frac{\sqrt{2}}{2}\sin\alpha & \cos\alpha & \frac{\sqrt{2}}{2}\sin\alpha
\end{bmatrix} \tag{7.2.14}
$$

From $H^{\mathrm{T}}H = \frac{4}{3}I_{3\times3}$ obtain the following equation set,

$$
\begin{cases}
1 + \frac{1}{2}\sin^2\alpha = 4/3 \\
1 + \cos^2\alpha = 4/3
\end{cases} \tag{7.2.15}
$$

Solve $\alpha = 54.74°$, the function of performance index without fault is

$$
F_p(4,0) = E_T(0) = \sqrt{\sum_{i=1}^{3}\sum_{j=1}^{4}M_{ij}^2} = \sqrt{\frac{5}{2}} \tag{7.2.16}
$$

In case the measurement assembly on any axis fails, according to Eq. (7.2.7), the function of performance index is

$$
F_P(4,1) = \sqrt{\frac{1}{4}\left(E_T^2(1) + E_T^2(2) + E_T^2(3) + E_T^2(4)\right)} = 2.4495 \tag{7.2.17}
$$

In terms of tw0 orthogonal two inclined and three orthogonal two-inclined configuration plan, the optimal mounting angle and optimum performance index are no longer derived repeatedly, statistic the optimized results in Table 7.1.

We can see from the chart the performance index of three orthogonal two inclined configuration plan in optimum configuration is superior to that of the three orthogonal one inclined and two orthogonal two inclined, which means the increase in number of inertial devices will improve the reliable performance of the system. However, the volume, weight, and cost of the system will also be increased. The engineering problem shall be dealt with case by case. What need to be pointed out is that since there are four configuration mounting angles for two-orthogonal two-inclined and three-orthogonal two-inclined, the contradictory equations should

Table 7.1 Statistics of optimized results for different configuration plans

Configuration plan	Optimal configuration without faults	Performance index without fault F_P	Optimal configuration for single-axis failure	Performance index for single-axis failure F_P
Three-orthogonal one-inclined position	$\alpha = 54.74°$	$F_P = 1.5811$	$\alpha = 54.74°$	$F_P = 2.4495$
Two-orthogonal two-inclined position	Four groups of optimum solutions. Among which, one group is $\alpha_1 = 65.91°$, $\alpha_2 = 114.09°$, $\beta_1 = 63.44°$, $\beta_2 = 116.57°$	$F_P = 1.5300$	Two groups of optimum solutions. Among which, one group is $\alpha_1 = 65.91°$, $\alpha_2 = 114.09°$, $\beta_1 = 63.44°$, $\beta_2 = 116.57°$	$F_P = 2.2225$
Three orthogonal two inclined position	Twenty-four groups of optimum solutions. Among which, one group is $\alpha_1 = 54.74°$, $\alpha_2 = 125.26°$, $\beta_1 = 45°$, $\beta_2 = 135°$	$F_P = 1.4243$	Twenty groups of optimum solutions. Among which, one group is $\alpha_1 = 54.74°$, $\alpha_2 = 125.26°$, $\beta_1 = 45°$, $\beta_2 = 135°$	$F_P = 1.7960$

be solved during the process of solving the optimum mounting angle, which is the reason that has multi groups of optimum solutions.

7.2.2 System-Level Redundant Configuration of Multi-inertial Group

In accordance with the difference of system structure and behaviors, the system-level strapdown redundancy may be divided into multi-strapdown backup redundancy, multi-strapdown voting redundancy, etc.

1. Multi Strapdown Backup Redundant Configuration

The multi-strapdown backup redundant configuration commonly has more identical strapdowns. In system operation, only strapdown output is selected by output selector, and the other strapdowns are taken for backup. The strapdown selected is called host strap and the ones that have not been chosen are called standby strapdown. When the host strapdown detects one fault, it stops output, which will be replaced by standby strapdown. According to the startup modes, the backup redundant systems are classified into hot backup, warm backup, and cold backup. Hot backup refers to that during the system operation, all the strapdowns operate the same mission simultaneously, the output selector only chooses one output of the strapdowns as the measurement output. When the operating strapdown stops because of fault, the output of other modules are selected for system output. Cold backup refers to that during the system operation, only one strapdown is working and other strapdowns are in power off state. When the operating strapdown stops because of fault, one of the other strapdowns will start. Warm backup is similar to the cold one. Among all the strapdowns, there is only one strapdown in working mode, however, other strapdowns are in power-on state. When the operating strapdown stops because of fault, one of the other strapdowns will take the place to keep on working.

With regard to the backup redundant system, the reliability and safety of the system rely on whether the fault occurring on the working strapdown could be detected correctly and the output selector is completely reliable.

2. **Multi-Strapdown Voting Redundant Configuration**

The multi-strapdown voting redundancy is composed of multi-strapdowns. When more than one half of components are normal among all the strapdowns, the system work can normally. Commonly, the multi-strapdown voting plan takes the odd and even parity equation as the criterion of fault difference. It locates the faulty inertial component by comparing the results of two differences.

The most common multi strapdown voting redundancy is the three strapdown voting redundancy, which are applied widely. Following, we will illustrate the working principle of three strapdown voting in details.

The structural diagram of three strapdown going redundancy refers to Fig. 7.7. The data measured by each set of strapdown inertial group include the angular velocities $\omega_x, \omega_y, \omega_z$ of the flight vehicle along the three axle and the apparent acceleration a_x, a_y and a_z along three directions.

The system-level redundancy of the three SIMUs may be formed by the mode of coaxial mounting of three sets of SIMUs. The main SIMU is for aiming and the other two SIMUs may determine the azimuth by relations of mounting position. The redundant plan of three SIMUs is normally designed in accordance with the principle of Fault-Work, Fault-Safety. It adopts the master–slave mode, that is, when the primary equipment is normal, it will be controlled by the primary equipment. If the primary equipment has fault while the slave unit is normal, it will switch to the other two sets of SIMUs in sequence, there is no sharing of measurement information of the master–slave unit.

Such structure is composed of three sets of common inertial measurement units on the flight vehicle. It is unnecessary to add additional discriminating unit. There are 18 signals formed by two groups of signals measured, plus the velocity signals and angular velocity signals, which are sent to rocket-borne computer for fault identification and isolation of faulty elements through software (Fig. 7.8).

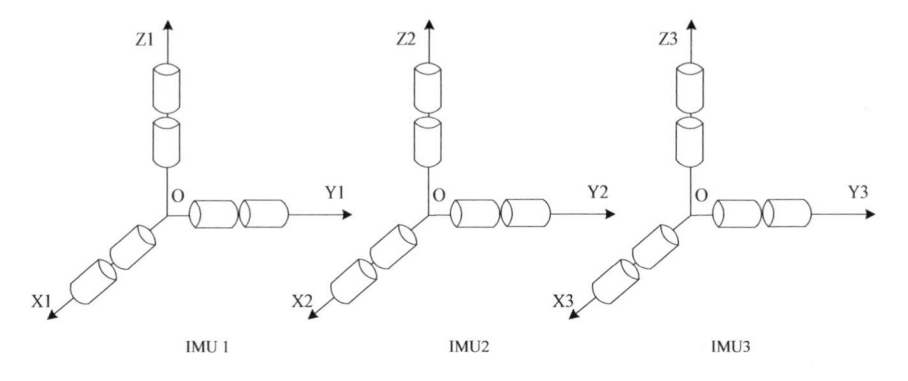

Fig. 7.7 Schematic diagram of coaxial mounting of three sets of IMU

Fig. 7.8 Three repeated redundant structures

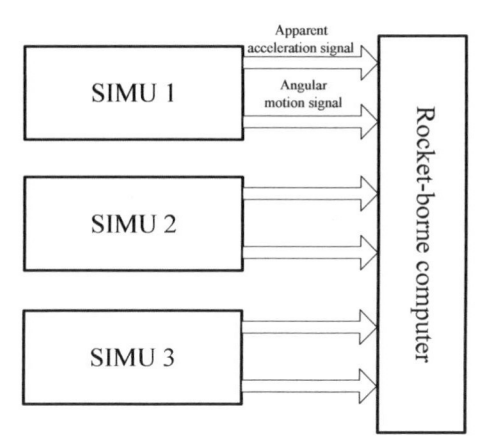

The fault identification of such structure adopts the voting criterion of the minority being subordinate to the majority. Two groups of measurement signals are needed to be identified: compare the two groups of signals of three sets of SIMUs respectively, the consistent one is that which has no fault. When one is inconsistent with the other two, such signal is the faulty signal. Among the six signals of each set of SIMU, any one or multi are identified as fault, such SIMU shall be judged as faulty.

Theoretically, for the measurement signal in the same quantity, if it has no fault, the measurement values shall be the same. However, gold cannot be pure and man cannot be perfect. Thus, the discriminant of apparent acceleration is

$$|a_{1J} - a_{2J}| \leq \varepsilon_{aJ} \tag{7.2.18}$$

$$|a_{2J} - a_{3J}| \leq \varepsilon_{aJ} \tag{7.2.19}$$

$$|a_{3J} - a_{1J}| \leq \varepsilon_{aJ} \tag{7.2.20}$$

Among which, the 1, 2 and 3 in following chart represent the number of inertial group, $J = x, y, z$ are the three directions.

The discriminant of attitude angle is

$$|\omega_{1J} - \omega_{2J}| \leq \varepsilon_{\omega J} \tag{7.2.21}$$

$$|\omega_{2J} - \omega_{3J}| \leq \varepsilon_{\omega J} \tag{7.2.22}$$

$$|\omega_{3J} - \omega_{1J}| \leq \varepsilon_{\omega J} \tag{7.2.23}$$

Here, 1, 2, and 3 are the number of the three SIMUs, ε_{aJ} and $\varepsilon_{\omega J}$ are the discriminant threshold of acceleration and angular velocity. If any of them is established, the other two will not be established. Then, the established one that does not include the SIMU is the faulty one. In identifying the above-mentioned six discriminants, it needs to integrate various types of possible errors and engineering factors to determine the value of the discriminant threshold. If the value of threshold is larger, the leakage probability is large. If it is small, the false identification is large. It needs to select the probability of leakage and false identification appropriately. The specific method to select threshold will be discussed in Sect. 8.3.2 in detail.

7.3   Fault Detection of Inertial Device

Fault detection of inertial devices contains testing and isolation. Detection is to detect the occurrence of fault. Isolation is to locate and remove the specific fault inertial device, to prevent the wrong measurement information from no longer being used by navigation system.

7.3.1   Fault Detection of Multi-table Fault for Single IMU

The fault detection and diagnosis of navigation system tend to adopt the state estimation method. The detecting way is to form residual serial with residual generator. The statistical analysis of residual serials could detect the occurrence of fault.

The redundant measurement equation formed by m inertial devices in the same precision. The measurement equation contains the function of noise interference. That is

$$Z = H\omega + \varepsilon \tag{7.3.1}$$

Here $\omega \in R^n$ is the system state to be detected. $Z \in R^m$ is the measurement value $(m > n)$ of m inertial devices. $H \in R^{m \times n}$ is the mounting matrix of device configuration, i.e., the column full rank matrices. ε is the Gaussian white noise sequence $\sigma^2 I_m$ of m-dimension zero-mean and covariance, i.e., $E(\varepsilon) = 0, E(\varepsilon\varepsilon^T) = \sigma^2 I_m, I_m$ is the m-order unit matrix.

The process of detecting fault of multi-table system of single IMU is the process of forming residual series through state estimation on the basis of measurement equation of inertial device, statistic characteristic difference of residual series under the comparison of fault and no fault, further identifying the occurrence of fault. The common methods consist of Generalized Likelihood Ratio Method (GLR), Singular Value Decomposition Method (SVO), Optimal Parity Vector Method, and statistical test method that needs mathematical model of system.

1. Generalized Likelihood Ratio Test (GLT)

GLT method is to separate the fault detection and isolation. The function of fault detection is the parity residuals of fault couple. The function of fault isolation is the statistical quantity of the maximum likelihoods function of related parity residuals under the assumption of various sensors being faulty.

Following parity equation is defined

$$P = VZ \tag{7.3.2}$$

Here, P is the parity vector, V is the row full rank matrix to be decided. Apparently, to have $P = VH\omega + V\varepsilon$ independent of the state to be measured ω and only related to noise or possible fault, let,

$$VH = 0, VV^T = I \tag{7.3.3}$$

Obtain,

$$P = V\varepsilon \tag{7.3.4}$$

When the gyroscope has no fault, the parity vector is only the function of noise. If fault occurs to the gyroscope, the measurement equation is changed to

$$Z = H\omega + b_f + \varepsilon \tag{7.3.5}$$

In it, b_f is the fault vector, which is corresponding to the disabled element zero. Other units are zero.

In like manner, obtain,

$$P = V\varepsilon + Vb_{\mathrm{f}} \tag{7.3.6}$$

At this moment, the parity vector not only relates to noise, but also related to fault. It is because that the inconsistency of parity vector with fault and no fault, provides reference for fault detection.

(1) Strategy of Fault Detection

The assumed examination of fault detection decision is as follows:
If no fault, the state $H_0 : E(P) = 0, E(PP^{\mathrm{T}}) = \sigma^2 VV^{\mathrm{T}} = \sigma^2$
If has fault, the State $H_1 : E(P) = \mu \neq 0, E((P - \mu)(P - \mu)^{\mathrm{T}}) = \sigma^2 VV^{\mathrm{T}} = \sigma^2$
In it, $\mu = Vb_{\mathrm{f}}$.
Since the parity vector P is the linear function of measuring noise ε, the P follows the Gaussian curve from m-n-dimensions. Under the situation of no fault and with fault, the likelihood functions are, respectively,

$$\varphi(P|H_0) = K \, \exp\left\{ -\frac{1}{2}\frac{p^{\mathrm{T}}p}{\sigma^2} \right\} \tag{7.3.7}$$

$$\varphi(P|H_1) = K \, exp\left\{ -\frac{1}{2}\frac{(p - \mu)^{\mathrm{T}}(p - \mu)}{\sigma^2} \right\} \tag{7.3.8}$$

Here $K = 1/\sqrt{(2\pi)^{m-n}\|V^{\mathrm{T}}V\|} \cdot \sigma$. The log-likelihood function formed from the above format is

$$L(P) = \ln\left[\frac{\varphi(P|H_1)}{\varphi(P|H_0)}\right] = \frac{1}{2}\left[\frac{P^{\mathrm{T}}P}{\sigma^2} - \frac{(P - \mu)^{\mathrm{T}}(P - \mu)}{\sigma^2}\right] \tag{7.3.9}$$

To solve μ in the format above, obtain the maximum likelihood estimation $\mu : \hat{\mu} = P$, the maximum likelihood estimator is

$$L_{\mathrm{max}}(P) = \frac{1}{2\sigma^2}\left[P^{\mathrm{T}}(VV^{\mathrm{T}})^{-1}P\right] = \frac{1}{2\sigma^2}\left[P^{\mathrm{T}}P\right] \tag{7.3.10}$$

Thus, P could be used for forming the fault detection decision function

$$\mathrm{FD_{GLT}} = \frac{1}{\sigma^2}\left[P^{\mathrm{T}}P\right] \tag{7.3.11}$$

Obviously, $\mathrm{FD_{GLT}} \sim \chi^2(m - n)$.
Therefore, the failure criterion is $\mathrm{FD_{GLT}} \geq T_D$, there is a fault. Otherwise, no fault occurs. Among which, T_D is to realize the given detection threshold.

(2) Fault Isolation and Fault Amplitude Estimation

The fault isolation includes m hypothesis testing. Let H_i is that the i sensor broke down, $E(P) = \mu_i \neq 0, E\left[(P - \mu_i)^{\mathrm{T}}(P - \mu_i)\right] = \sigma^2$. Here, $\mu_i = V^{\mathrm{T}}e_i f_i, e_i$ is m-dimension column vector that the i element is 1, and the other elements are 0. $V^{\mathrm{T}}e_i \overset{\Delta}{=} V_i^*$ is written as the transposed vector of the i row vector of the parity matrix V.

The log-likelihood function corresponding to the i sensor is

$$
\begin{aligned}
\ln[\varphi(p|H_i)] &= \ln K - \frac{1}{2}(p - \mu_i)^{\mathrm{T}} \frac{(V^{\mathrm{T}}V)^{-1}}{\sigma^2}(p - \mu_i) \\
&= \ln K - \frac{1}{2}(p - V_i^* f_i)^{\mathrm{T}} \frac{(V^{\mathrm{T}}V)^{-1}}{\sigma^2}(p - V_i^* f_i) \\
&= \ln K - \frac{1}{2}\left[\left(p^{\mathrm{T}} \frac{(V^{\mathrm{T}}V)^{-1}}{\sigma^2} p\right) - 2f\left(p^{\mathrm{T}} \frac{(V^{\mathrm{T}}V)^{-1}}{\sigma^2} V_i^*\right)\right. \\
&\quad \left. + f_i^*\left((V_i^*)^{\mathrm{T}} \frac{(V^{\mathrm{T}}V)^{-1}}{\sigma^2} V_i^*\right)\right]
\end{aligned}
$$

As for solving derivative of f_i in the formula above, obtain the maximum likelihood estimation f_i,

$$
\hat{f} = \frac{p^{\mathrm{T}}(V^{\mathrm{T}}V)^{-1}V_i^*}{(V_i^*)^{\mathrm{T}}(V^{\mathrm{T}}V)^{-1}V_i^*} \tag{7.3.12}
$$

The maximum likelihood estimator is

$$
\ln[\varphi(p|H_i)]_{\max} = \ln K - \frac{1}{2}p^{\mathrm{T}} \frac{(V^{\mathrm{T}}V)^{-1}}{\sigma^2}p + \frac{1}{2}\frac{\left[p^{\mathrm{T}}(V^{\mathrm{T}}V)^{-1}V_i^*\right]^2}{\sigma^2(V_i^*)^{\mathrm{T}}(V^{\mathrm{T}}V)^{-1}V_i^*} \tag{7.3.13}
$$

Notice that $V^{\mathrm{T}}V = I_{m-n}$, the decision function of fault isolation determined by the formula above is

$$
\mathrm{FI}_{\mathrm{GLT}}(i) = \frac{1}{\sigma^2}\frac{\left[p^{\mathrm{T}}(V^{\mathrm{T}}V)^{-1}V_i^*\right]^2}{(V_i^*)^{\mathrm{T}}(V^{\mathrm{T}}V)^{-1}V_i^*} = \frac{1}{\sigma^2}\frac{(p^{\mathrm{T}}V_i^*)^2}{(V_i^*)^{\mathrm{T}}V_i^*} \tag{7.3.14}
$$

If the larger $\mathrm{FI}_{\mathrm{GLT}}(i)$ is, the larger $\ln[\varphi(p|H_i)]_{\max}$ is obtained . It means that the probability of the i sensor going wrong is larger.

If the isolation function value of the k sensor is the maximum value among all the isolation function values of the sensors, that is,

$$\text{FI}_{\text{GLT}}(k) = \max_{1 \leq i \leq m} \{\text{FI}_{\text{GLT}}(i)\} \qquad (7.3.15)$$

The k sensor is judged as faulty.

2. Singular Value Decomposition Method (SVD)

From configuration matrix $H \in R^{m \times n}$, and given rank$H = r$, it is known that the singular value decomposition is

$$U^*HV = \Lambda = \begin{bmatrix} \Sigma & 0 \\ 0 & 0 \end{bmatrix}, \quad H = UHV^* = U\begin{bmatrix} \Sigma & 0 \\ 0 & 0 \end{bmatrix}V^* \qquad (7.3.16)$$

In it, $UU^* \approx U^*U = I_m, VV^* = V^*V = I_n, \sum = \text{diag}\{\lambda_1, \lambda_2, \ldots, \lambda_r\}$. U is further decomposed as $U = [U_1 : U_2], \Lambda = [\Sigma \quad 0]^{\text{T}}; V = I_m$. When the system has fault, the equations at two sides are

$$Z = HX + b_{\text{f}} + \varepsilon \qquad (7.3.17)$$

Here, b_{f} is the fault vector, the unit of the related fault sensor is not zero. Other units are zero.

Put the above-decomposed equation into the one at the two sides of fault system, and obtain,

$$Z = U\Lambda V^*X + b_{\text{f}} + \varepsilon \qquad (7.3.18)$$

The left end times U^* and obtain, $U^*Z = \Lambda V^*X + U^*b_{\text{f}} + U^*\varepsilon$, decompose it as

$$\begin{cases} U_1^*Z = \sum VX + U_1^*(b_{\text{f}} + \varepsilon) \\ U_2^*Z = U_2^*b_{\text{f}} + U_2^*\varepsilon \end{cases} \qquad (7.3.19)$$

Form the parity vector $P = U_2U_2^*Z = U_2U_2^*(b_{\text{f}} + \varepsilon)$. Then, the parity vector has nothing to do with the state vector. When the system goes wrong, the parity vector is not only the function of noise, but also the function of fault. It is the inconsistency of the parity vector between with fault and without fault, the fault diagnosis could be fulfilled. The SVD method realizes the fault detection according to the fault detection and isolation function of parity vector in different principles. Such method could not only detect the fault of single gyroscope, but also the situation that two gyroscopes become fault. The specific algorithm is as follows:

(1) Calculate U_2 from configuration matrix H;
(2) Calculate the reference vector $f_1, f_2, \ldots, f_i$ when one or two gyroscopes broke down simultaneously,
(3) $k = \text{argmax}(P^{\text{T}}f_i)$;
(4) $\text{DFD}_k = P^{\text{T}}f_k$; If $P^{\text{T}}f_k > TD$, then the k gyroscope becomes fault. Otherwise, it works normally. TD is the detection threshold.

(5) Fault reference vector is defined as $f_i = \dfrac{\mathrm{col}_i(U_2 U_2^*)}{\|\mathrm{col}_i(U_2 U_2^*)\|}$. Here, $\mathrm{col}_i()$ shows the column i.

3. Optimal Parity Vector Method (OPT)

OPT Method is to carry out fault detection and fault isolation simultaneously. Design the optimal parity vector that is sensitive to particular sensor instead of the faults of other sensors and the measured noise according to one type of performance index function. Then, calculate the parity residual of various redundant sensors. Select the maximum absolute values or maximum squared value of these parity residuals for fault detection and isolation.

Consider the common measurement equation

$$Z = H\omega + Db_f + F\varepsilon \tag{7.3.20}$$

D and F are the respective fault input matrix and noise input matrix. To design the parity vector that is sensitive to the fault of particular sensor, set up the performance index function as follows:

$$
\begin{aligned}
S_i &= \max \frac{(v_i^\mathrm{T} De_i)^2}{\|v_i^\mathrm{T} F\|^2 + \sum_{j \neq i}(v_i^\mathrm{T} De_j)^2} \\
&= \max \frac{(v_i^\mathrm{T} De_i)^2}{v_i^\mathrm{T}(FF^\mathrm{T} + \sum_{j \neq i} De_j e_j^\mathrm{T} D^\mathrm{T})v_i}, \quad VH = 0
\end{aligned}
\tag{7.3.21}
$$

Here, $\|v_i^\mathrm{T} F\|$ is the model of vector $v_i^\mathrm{T} F$, e_i and v_i are the i row vector of I_m and the optimal parity vector of fault detection of the i sensor to be designed. $v_i^\mathrm{T} De_i$ and $v_i^\mathrm{T} De_j$ show the sensitivity for the fault of the i and the j sensors, while $\|v_i^\mathrm{T} F\|$ shows the noise sensitivity. The numerator shows the measure of fault sensitivity of the sensor measured, the denominator shows the measure of sensitivity of the faults of other sensors and all the noise. In addition, the odd even constraint is kept.

In considering the odd–even constraint, the parity vector v_i could be shown in the linear combination $v_i = V^\mathrm{T} c_i$ of V, and put into Formula (7.3.21), it reaches the maximum at the place of $c_i = a M_{Bi}^{-1} u_i$.

In it, a is the arbitrary real number, $u_i = VDe_i \in R^{m-n}$; $M_{Bi} = V(FF^\mathrm{T} + DD^\mathrm{T} - De_i e_i^\mathrm{T} D^\mathrm{T})V^\mathrm{T}$ is the $m - n$ order symmetric matrices.

Then, the vector v_i to be solved is the optimum parity vector, and given by following format:

$$v_i = V^\mathrm{T} c_i = a V^\mathrm{T} M_{Bi}^{-1} u_i \tag{7.3.22}$$

Without loss of generality, put v_i in unitization, and obtain the optimum parity vector $v_i^* = v_i/\|v_i\|$. Thus, use v_i^* to detect whether the i sensor has fault or not. For convenience, the optimum parity vector v_i^* is in unitization with v_i . Then, the corresponding optimal parity residuals is $d_i^* = v_i^T Z$. If $b_f = 0$, then, $d_i^* \sim N(0, \sigma^2 \|v_i^T F\|^2)$. The decision function of fault detection is the standard statistics of d_i^*.

$$d_i = d_i^* / (\sigma \|v_i^T F\|) \tag{7.3.23}$$

Given false alarm rate T, find the $1 - T/2$ quantile in standardized normal distribution, obtain the fault detection threshold $T_D = u_1 - T/2$. Calculate the maximum absolute in d_i : $|d_k| = \max_i |d_i|$. If $|d_k| > T_D$, the k sensor is judged as fault. Otherwise, no fault is judged.

It can be seen from the above-mentioned process, actually, the OPT equation is to combine the processes of fault detection and isolation together and carry out simultaneously. If fault is detected, it is certain that the fault is isolated.

7.3.2 System-Level Fault Detection of Multi-IMUs

This section discusses the design of fault detection plan on the basis of three strapdown voting redundant plans mentioned in Sect. 7.2.2. Among the three strapdown redundant plans, the three sets of SIMUs are installed by sharing the support and reference in the same azimuth. The diagnosis of coaxality fault mainly has three methods, voting method, parity equation method, and mean value test. Here, the voting method algorithm is the simple one, because it is easy to determine the threshold, and sensitive to fault, with quick diagnosis. Thus, the voting method is used for fault detection.

Among the three strapdown redundant plans, each physical quantity (such as acceleration, angular velocity) to be measured has three sensors to be measured simultaneously. Therefore, in actual diagnosis, we shall subtract the output of two numbers of the three sensors and take the absolute values, and obtain the absolutes of two numbers of the three groups. If the difference of two groups is larger and one is small, it means the difference of the output of one sensor with the other two is larger, naturally, such sensor could be regarded as faulty. The two sensors with less difference work normally, and the output is credible. If the differences of three groups are large, the coaxial double fault occurs, the outputs of three sensors are unconvincing, the voting method becomes invalid. It needs to diagnose the coaxial double fault with other methods. If the differences of two groups among the three are small, and only one group is larger, the output of two sensors related to the larger difference is normal, and it is just at the two sides of the truth-value, the three sensors work normally.

1. Specific Flow of Voting Algorithm

   (1) Assuming that the outputs of the three sensors of the same physical quantity are respectively x_1, x_2, x_3, subtract the two numbers and take the absolute values, let $z_1 = |x_1 - x_2|, z_2 = |x_1 - x_3|, z_3 = |x_2 - x_3|$;

   (2) Take one threshold T_D (the specific decision method refers to Sect. 7.3.2, compare z_1, z_2, z_3 with T_D;

   (3) If z_1, z_2, z_3 are smaller than T_D, the three sensors are judged as working normally, the three outputs are valid. In calculating navigation, take the average of the three numbers as the input.

   (4) If two of z_1, z_2 and z_3 are smaller than T_D, one is larger than T_D, then, the three sensors are judged normal. The input in calculating navigation could also take the average of the three numbers as the output.

   (5) If two of z_1, z_2 and z_3 are larger than T_D, one is smaller than T_D, then, one sensor is taken as fault, the two sensors whose difference less than T_D have no fault. The input in calculating navigation will take the average of the output of the two sensors without fault.

   (6) If all the z_1, z_2 and z_3 are larger than T_D, find the largest two from them and the difference of the remaining group is regarded as less, these two sensors have no fault. The calculation of navigation will take the average of the output of such two sensors as the input.

2. Threshold Definite Method

Restricted by the space, this section only discusses the threshold definite method under the condition of pure noise. First, the definition of mistake rate and miss rate are introduced.

In fault detection, H_0 means no fault, H_1 shows have fault. There are four types of possibilities [7]

(1) H_0 is true, take H_1 as the true, this is called detection error, its probability is written as P_F;

(2) H_1 is true, H_0 is judged as true, this is called missed detection, its probability is written as P_M;

(3) H_0 is true, and H_0 is judged as true, this is called no error detection, its probability is written as $1 - P_F$;

(4) H_1 is true, H_1 is judged as true, this is called correct detection, its probability is written as $P_D = 1 - P_M$;

The error detection rate may be defined as

$$P_F = P(\text{judges} H_1 \text{true} | H_0 \text{true})$$

The undetected error rate may be defined as

$$P_M = P(\text{Judge}H_0\text{true}|H_1\text{true})$$

The outputs of the three coaxial-mounted sensors at certain moment are x_1, x_2 and x_3, respectively, the true physical quantity of the three sensors measured at the moment is x, the measured noise is the zero-mean white noise with the variance σ_n, shown with w, then,

$$x_1 = x + w_1 \tag{7.3.24}$$

$$x_2 = x + w_2 \tag{7.3.25}$$

$$x_3 = x + w_3 \tag{7.3.26}$$

Here, $w_1, w_2, w_3 \sim N(0, \sigma_n^2)$, and w_1, w_2 and w_3 are independent mutually,

$$x_1 - x_2 = w_1 - w_2 \tag{7.3.27}$$

$$x_1 - x_3 = w_1 - w_3 \tag{7.3.28}$$

$$x_2 - x_3 = w_1 - w_2 \tag{7.3.29}$$

Since $w_1, w_2, w_3 \sim N(0, \sigma_n^2)$, and w_1, w_2, w_3 are independent mutually, therefore, $(w_1 - w_2), (w_1 - w_3), (w_2 - w_3) \sim N(0, 2\sigma_n^2)$.   Thus, $(x_1 - x_2), (x_1 - x_3)$, $(x_2 - x_3) \sim N(0, 2\sigma_n^2)$,

Given there is event

$$A_1 : |x_1 - x_2| < T_{Dn}$$
$$A_2 : |x_1 - x_3| < T_{Dn}$$
$$A_3 : |x_2 - x_3| < T_{Dn}$$

Given the false alarm rate is α, then, m $P(\text{Judge}H_1\text{true}|H_0\text{true}) = \alpha$. The threshold is T_{D_n}, the condition of judging H_0 true conditions A_1A_2, A_3 have two happening simultaneously. The probability of Event A_i ($i = 1, 2, 3$) occurrence is $(1 - \lambda)$, at this moment, use binary system 0 to represent the occurrence of Event A_i ($i = 1, 2, 3$), the binary system 1 shows the nonoccurrence of Event A_i ($i = 1, 2, 3$), the occurrence refers to following table:

From the table above, we could know that the probability of simultaneous occurrence of more than two events A_i ($i = 1, 2, 3$) is

$$\lambda^3 + 3\lambda^2(1 - \lambda) = 1 - \alpha \tag{7.3.30}$$

Again because λ is the probability of event occurrence, the $0 \leq \lambda \leq 1$ is permanently established. Solve Eq. (2.3.7) and based on such condition $0 \leq \lambda \leq 1$ then, the final value of λ could be obtained.

Table 7.2 The occurrence and corresponding probability of event A_i ($i = 1, 2, 3$)

No.	Event occurrence	Probability of occurrence
000	A_1 occur A_2 occur A_3 occur	$(1 - \lambda)^3$
001	A_1 occur A_2 occur A_3 nonoccurrence	$\lambda(1 - \lambda)^2$
010	A_1 occur A_2 nonoccurrence A_3 occur	$\lambda(1 - \lambda)^2$
011	A_1 occur A_2 nonoccurrence A_3 nonoccurrence	$\lambda^2(1 - \lambda)$
100	A_1 nonoccurrence A_2 occur A_3 occur	$\lambda(1 - \lambda)^2$
101	A_1 nonoccurrence A_2 occur A_3 nonoccurrence	$\lambda^2(1 - \lambda)$
110	A_1 nonoccurrence A_2 nonoccurrence A_3 occur	$\lambda^2(1 - \lambda)$
111	A_1 nonoccurrence A_2 nonoccurrence A_3 nonoccurrence	λ^3

$$T_{Dn} = z_{(1-\lambda/2)} * \sqrt{2}\sigma_n \qquad (7.3.31)$$

In it, $z_{(1-\lambda/2)}$ quantile of the standardized normal distribution $(1 - \lambda/2)$. Since only noise is considered, hence,

$$T_D = T_{Dn} \qquad (7.3.32)$$

It is worth mentioning that the probability of occurrence in Table 7.2 is not so accurate, because z_1, z_2 and z_3 are not independent mutually, there is one issue of correlation. However, the output noise of the three sensors are independent, the difference of the two numbers could be approximately taken as independent.

7.4 Fault Reconfiguration of Inertial Devices

After detecting the fault device, the mission is to isolate the fault device, and organize the remaining normal devices to provide correct information of measurement. As for the multi-table redundant system of single inertial group, the fault isolation is to delete the rows corresponding to the fault device for processing. This is equal to isolate the fault device. The process of fault reconfiguration is to apply the remaining normal inertial devices, and reconfigure and process the remaining information of measurement through related principles of data fusion to obtain the necessary measurement quantity. With regard to the system-level redundancy of multi-inertial groups, fault isolation is to remove the fault inertial devices detected from the information of measurement. Fault reconfiguration is to select the appropriate sensors as the output of measurement information from the remaining normal sensors.

7.4.1 *Multi-table Fault Reconfiguration of Single IMU*

Due to the existence of measurement matrix, while reconfiguring data for multi-table redundant system of single IMU, the least square method is emphasized.

1. Fault Reconfiguration of the Least Square Method

The index of the least square estimation is to minimize the quadratic sum of the difference between the measurement Z and the estimated $\hat{Z} = H\hat{X}$ of the measurement determined by $\hat{X}$, that is,

$$\min J(\hat{X}) = \min(Z - H\hat{\omega})^{\mathrm{T}}(Z - H\hat{\omega}) \tag{7.4.1}$$

To minimize the formula above, it should meet

$$\frac{\partial J(\hat{X})}{\partial X} = -2H^{\mathrm{T}}(Z - H\hat{X}) = 0 \tag{7.4.2}$$

If H has the maximum rank n, that is $H^T H$ positive definite, and $m > n$, the least square estimation X is

$$\hat{X} = (H^{\mathrm{T}}H)^{-1}H^{\mathrm{T}}Z \tag{7.4.3}$$

If the measured noise ε is the random vector with mean zero and variance R, the mean square error matrix estimated by least square at this moment is

$$E[\tilde{X}\tilde{X}^{\mathrm{T}}] = (H^{\mathrm{T}}H)^{-1}H^{\mathrm{T}}RH(H^{\mathrm{T}}H)^{-1} \tag{7.4.4}$$

The least square estimation applies the information of measurement regardless of good or not, in the multi-table inertial devices redundant configuration plan, since the accuracy of inertial devices in orthogonal installation and inclined installation are different, the accuracy of measurement is also varied. Thus, the weighted least square method may be used for fault reconfiguration. The weighting of measurement information of orthogonal axis with high accuracy shall be taken larger, and the weighting of measurement information of inclined axis with poor accuracy shall be taken less. The solving criteria of estimating weighted least square is

$$J(\hat{X}) = (Z - H\hat{\omega})^{\mathrm{T}}W(Z - H\hat{\omega}) = \min \tag{7.4.5}$$

Solution,

$$\hat{X} = [H^{\mathrm{T}}(W + W^{\mathrm{T}})H]^{-1}H^{\mathrm{T}}(W + W^{\mathrm{T}})Z \tag{7.4.6}$$

Commonly, the weighted matrix takes symmetric matrix, that is $W = W^T$. Thus, the weighted least square estimation at this moment is

$$\hat{X} = (H^T W H)^{-1} H^T W Z \tag{7.4.7}$$

The estimated error is

$$
\begin{aligned}
\tilde{X} = X - \hat{X} &= (H^T W H)^{-1} H^T W H X - (H^T W H)^{-1} H^T W Z \\
&= (H^T W H)^{-1} H^T W (H X - Z) = -(H^T W H)^{-1} H^T W V
\end{aligned}
\tag{7.4.8}
$$

If the mean value of the measured error ε is zero, covariance matrix is R, by then, the weighted least square is estimated as unbiased estimate. The estimated mean square deviation is

$$
\begin{aligned}
E[\tilde{X}\tilde{X}^T] &= E\left[(H^T W H)^{-1} H^T W V \left((H^T W H)^{-1} H^T W V \right)^T \right] \\
&= E\left[(H^T W H)^{-1} H^T W V V^T W^T H (H^T W H)^{-1} \right] \\
&= (H^T W H)^{-1} H^T W R W^T H (H^T W H)^{-1}
\end{aligned}
\tag{7.4.9}
$$

When $W = R^{-1}$, the estimated mean square error is smaller than that of any other weighted least square estimation, therefore, the estimated one when $W = R^{-1}$ is the optimum one in weighted least square estimation. At this moment, the weighted least square estimation is

$$\hat{X} = (H^T R^{-1} H)^{-1} H^T R^{-1} Z \tag{7.4.10}$$

The mean square error estimated is

$$E[\tilde{X}\tilde{X}^T] = (H^T R^{-1} H)^{-1} \tag{7.4.11}$$

Following, take the three orthogonal one inclined eight table installation scheme in Sect. 7.2.1 as the example, discuss the correctness of the least square estimation and weighted least square estimation. The configuration plan refers to Fig. 7.2. At this moment, the mounting angle $\alpha = 54.74°$, the variance of the measurement error of orthogonal devices is σ^2, the measurement error of inclined device is $25\sigma^2$. By then the installation matrix is

$$H = \begin{bmatrix} 1 & 0 & 0 \\ 0 & 1 & 0 \\ 0 & 0 & 1 \\ \frac{\sqrt{2}}{2}\sin\alpha & \frac{\sqrt{2}}{2}\sin\alpha & \cos\alpha \end{bmatrix} \qquad (7.4.12)$$

Under the situation of no fault, the module of estimated mean square error obtained by the least square method is

$$\left\| E\big[\tilde{X}\tilde{X}^{\mathrm{T}}\big] \right\| = \left\| (H^{\mathrm{T}}H)^{-1}H^{\mathrm{T}}RH(H^{\mathrm{T}}H)^{-1} \right\| = 6.652\sigma^2 \qquad (7.4.13)$$

The module of estimated mean square error obtained by the weighted least square method is

$$\left\| E\big[\tilde{X}\tilde{X}^{\mathrm{T}}\big] \right\| = \left\| (H^{\mathrm{T}}R^{-1}H)^{-1} \right\| = 1.710\sigma^2 \qquad (7.4.14)$$

From the results we can see that, when considers the different installation accuracy of orthogonal axle and inclined axis, the estimated error by the weighted least square method is smaller, the accuracy of estimation is higher.

2. Three-orthogonal multi-inclined fault reconfiguration

The three-orthogonal multi-inclined redundant scheme refers to Fig. 7.9. The X, Y, Z are the three mutually orthogonal axes. In the $OXYZ$ three-dimensional space, there are N inclined axes. The included angle of inclined axes with the X, Y, Z axle are the respective $\alpha_1, \ldots, \alpha_N, \beta_1, \ldots, \beta_N, \gamma_1, \ldots, \gamma_N$.

Fig. 7.9 Three-orthogonal multi-inclined installation diagram

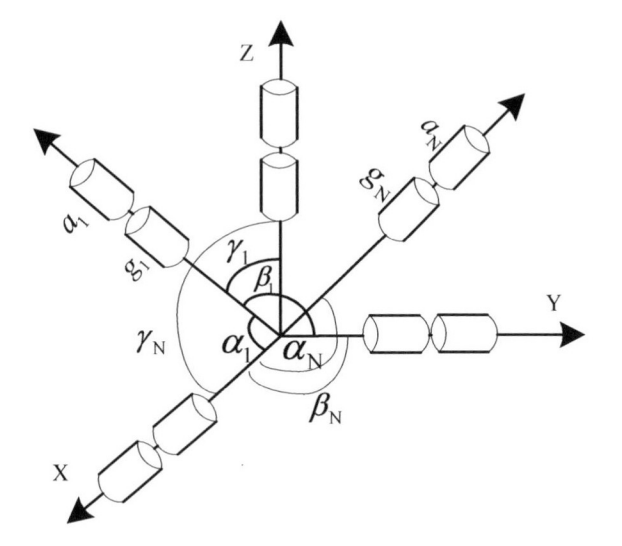

The installation matrix of the system is

$$H = \begin{bmatrix} 1 & 0 & 0 \\ 0 & 1 & 0 \\ 0 & 0 & 1 \\ \cos\alpha_1 & \cos\beta_1 & \cos\gamma_1 \\ \vdots & \vdots & \vdots \\ \cos\alpha_N & \cos\beta_N & \cos\gamma_N \end{bmatrix} \tag{7.4.15}$$

Because the system does not require to reconfigure when inclined axle is fault, it only outputs the measured value of the inertial devices on orthogonal axes. The device on orthogonal axis X, and the angular velocities in three directions are ω_x, ω_y and ω_z. The measurement output on the five axes are the respectively $m_X, m_Y, m_Z, m_1 \ldots m_N$. When the device on orthogonal axis X goes wrong, the installation matrix is changed as

$$\begin{bmatrix} m_Y \\ m_Z \\ m_1 \\ \vdots \\ m_N \end{bmatrix} = \begin{bmatrix} 0 & 1 & 0 \\ 0 & 0 & 1 \\ \cos\alpha_1 & \cos\beta_1 & \cos\gamma_1 \\ \vdots & \vdots & \vdots \\ \cos\alpha_N & \cos\beta_N & \cos\gamma_N \end{bmatrix} \begin{bmatrix} \omega_x \\ \omega_y \\ \omega_z \end{bmatrix} \tag{7.4.16}$$

Expand the matrix

$$\begin{cases} \hat{\omega}_{x1} = \dfrac{m_1 - m_Y \cos\beta_1 - m_Z \cos\gamma_1}{\cos\alpha_1} \\ \quad\vdots \\ \hat{\omega}_{xN} = \dfrac{m_N - m_Y \cos\beta_N - m_Z \cos\gamma_N}{\cos\alpha_N} \end{cases} \tag{7.4.17}$$

Here, $\hat{\omega}_{xN}$ shows the reconfiguration value of X-axis obtained from Y, Z, g_N axle. Then, $\hat{\omega}_x = k_1 \cdot \hat{\omega}_{x1} + \cdots + k_N \cdot \hat{\omega}_{xN}$. The weighting coefficients $k_1, k_2, \ldots, k_N$ have the following constrained conditions,

$$\begin{cases} k_1 + k_2 + \cdots + k_N = 1 \\ \dfrac{k_1}{k_N} = \dfrac{|\cos\alpha_1|}{|\cos\alpha_N|} \end{cases} \tag{7.4.18}$$

The following is obtained:

$$
\begin{aligned}
\hat{\omega}_x &= k_1 \cdot \hat{\omega}_{x1} + \cdots + k_N \cdot \hat{\omega}_{xN} \\
&= \frac{|\cos\alpha_1|}{\sum\limits_{i=1}^{N}|\cos\alpha_i|} \cdot \hat{\omega}_{x1} + \frac{|\cos\alpha_2|}{\sum\limits_{i=1}^{N}|\cos\alpha_i|} \cdot \hat{\omega}_{x2} + \cdots + \frac{|\cos\alpha_N|}{\sum\limits_{i=1}^{N}|\cos\alpha_i|} \cdot \hat{\omega}_{xN} \\
&= \frac{|\cos\alpha_1|}{\sum\limits_{i=1}^{N}|\cos\alpha_i|} \cdot \frac{m_1 - m_Y\cos\beta_1 - m_Z\cos\gamma_1}{\cos\alpha_1} \\
&\quad + \cdots \frac{|\cos\alpha_N|}{\sum\limits_{i=1}^{N}|\cos\alpha_i|} \cdot \frac{m_N - m_Y\cos\beta_N - m_Z\cos\gamma_N}{\cos\alpha_N} \\
&= \frac{sign(\cos\alpha_1)\cdot(m_1 - m_Y\cos\beta_1 - m_Z\cos\gamma_1)}{\sum\limits_{i=1}^{N}|\cos\alpha_i|} + \cdots \\
&\quad + \frac{sign(\cos\alpha_N)\cdot(m_N - m_Y\cos\beta_N - m_Z\cos\gamma_N)}{\sum\limits_{i=1}^{N}|\cos\alpha_i|} \\
&= \sum_{j=1}^{N} \frac{sign(\cos\alpha_j)\cdot(m_j - m_Y\cos\beta_j - m_Z\cos\gamma_j)}{\sum\limits_{i=1}^{N}|\cos\alpha_i|}
\end{aligned}
\tag{7.4.19}
$$

In the same manner, the following is obtained:
When the device on orthogonal axis Y goes wrong

$$
\hat{\omega}_y = \sum_{j=1}^{N} \frac{sign(\cos\beta_j)\cdot(m_j - m_X\cos\alpha_j - m_Z\cos\gamma_j)}{\sum\limits_{i=1}^{N}|\cos\beta_i|}
\tag{7.4.20}
$$

When the device on orthogonal axis Z goes wrong,

$$
\hat{\omega}_z = \sum_{j=1}^{N} \frac{sign(\cos\gamma_j)\cdot(m_j - m_X\cos\alpha_j - m_Y\cos\beta_j)}{\sum\limits_{i=1}^{N}|\cos\gamma_i|}
\tag{7.4.21}
$$

Equations (7.4.19–7.4.21) present the reconfiguration strategy with the most data of reconfigured devices, that is, to use all the redundant devices for reconfiguration, also may use partial redundant devices for reconfiguration. Different reconfiguration strategies used may have different accuracy of reconfiguration.

3. Numerical Examples

The three-orthogonal two-inclined configuration scheme in Fig. 7.6 is an example to illustrate the process and accuracy of reconfiguration. The configuration angles of the inclined axes g_1 and $g_2 \alpha_1 = 125.9°, \beta_1 = 46.6°, \gamma_1 = 115.4°, \alpha_2 = 46.5°, \beta_2 = 56.5°, \gamma_2 = 118°$, the installation accuracy of orthogonal axis and inclined axes are the same as above, which are σ^2 and $25\sigma^2$ respectively. If the device on orthogonal axis X goes wrong,

(1) Apply orthogonal axle Y, Z and inclined axis g_1 for fault reconfiguration for orthogonal axis X, the measurement matrix is

$$\begin{bmatrix} m_Y \\ m_Z \\ m_1 \end{bmatrix} = \begin{bmatrix} 0 & 1 & 0 \\ 0 & 0 & 1 \\ \cos \alpha_1 & \cos \beta_1 & \cos \gamma_1 \end{bmatrix} \begin{bmatrix} \omega_x \\ \omega_y \\ \omega_z \end{bmatrix} \qquad (7.4.22)$$

Hence,

$$\hat{\omega}_x = \frac{m_1 - 0.6871 \cdot m_Y + 0.4289 \cdot m_Z}{-0.5864} \qquad (7.4.23)$$

To solve the variance of reconfiguration error with the weighted least square method,

$$D(\hat{\omega}_x) = \left\| (H^T R^{-1} H)^{-1} \right\| = 74.657\sigma^2 \qquad (7.4.24)$$

(2) Apply the orthogonal axes Y and Z and inclined axis g_2 for fault reconfiguration of orthogonal axis X, the measurement matrix is

$$\begin{bmatrix} m_Y \\ m_Z \\ m_2 \end{bmatrix} = \begin{bmatrix} 0 & 1 & 0 \\ 0 & 0 & 1 \\ \cos \alpha_2 & \cos \beta_2 & \cos \gamma_2 \end{bmatrix} \begin{bmatrix} \omega_x \\ \omega_y \\ \omega_z \end{bmatrix} \qquad (7.4.25)$$

Hence

$$\hat{\omega}_x = \frac{m_2 - 0.6871 \cdot m_Y + 0.4289 \cdot m_Z}{-0.5864} \qquad (7.4.26)$$

To solve the variance of reconfiguration error with the weighted least square method,

$$D(\hat{\omega}_x) = \left\| (H^T R^{-1} H)^{-1} \right\| = 53.906\sigma^2 \qquad (7.4.27)$$

(3) Apply the orthogonal axis Y and inclined axes g_1, g_2 for fault reconfiguration of orthogonal axis X, the measurement matrix is

$$\begin{bmatrix} m_Y \\ m_1 \\ m_2 \end{bmatrix} = \begin{bmatrix} 0 & 1 & 0 \\ \cos \alpha_1 & \cos \beta_1 & \cos \gamma_1 \\ \cos \alpha_2 & \cos \beta_2 & \cos \gamma_2 \end{bmatrix} \begin{bmatrix} \omega_x \\ \omega_y \\ \omega_z \end{bmatrix} \tag{7.4.28}$$

Hence

$$\hat{\omega}_x = \frac{\cos \gamma_2 \cdot m_1 - \cos \beta_1 \cdot \cos \gamma_2 \cdot m_Y - \cos \gamma_1 \cdot m_2 + \cos \gamma_1 \cos \beta_2 \cdot m_Z}{\cos \alpha_1 \cos \gamma_2 - \cos \alpha_2 \cos \gamma_1} \tag{7.4.29}$$

To solve the variance of reconfiguration error with the weighted least square method,

$$D(\hat{\omega}_x) = \left\| (H^T R^{-1} H)^{-1} \right\| = 72.306\sigma^2 \tag{7.4.30}$$

(4) Apply the orthogonal axis Z and inclined axes g_1, g_2 for fault reconfiguration of orthogonal axis X, the measurement matrix is

$$\begin{bmatrix} m_Z \\ m_1 \\ m_2 \end{bmatrix} = \begin{bmatrix} 0 & 0 & 1 \\ \cos \alpha_1 & \cos \beta_1 & \cos \gamma_1 \\ \cos \alpha_2 & \cos \beta_2 & \cos \gamma_2 \end{bmatrix} \begin{bmatrix} \omega_x \\ \omega_y \\ \omega_z \end{bmatrix} \tag{7.4.31}$$

Hence,

$$\hat{\omega}_x = \frac{\cos \beta_2 \cdot m_1 - \cos \gamma_1 \cdot \cos \beta_2 \cdot m_Z - \cos \beta_1 \cdot m_2 + \cos \beta_1 \cos \gamma_2 \cdot m_Z}{\cos \alpha_1 \cos \beta_2 - \cos \alpha_2 \cos \beta_1}$$

$$\tag{7.4.32}$$

To solve the variance of reconfiguration error with the weighted least square method,

$$D(\hat{\omega}_x) = \left\| (H^T R^{-1} H)^{-1} \right\| = 44.856\sigma^2 \tag{7.4.33}$$

(5) Apply orthogonal axes Y and Z and inclined axes g_1, g_2 for fault reconfiguration of orthogonal axis X, the measurement matrix is

$$\begin{bmatrix} m_Y \\ m_Z \\ m_1 \\ m_2 \end{bmatrix} = \begin{bmatrix} 0 & 1 & 0 \\ 0 & 0 & 1 \\ \cos \alpha_1 & \cos \beta_1 & \cos \gamma_1 \\ \cos \alpha_2 & \cos \beta_2 & \cos \gamma_2 \end{bmatrix} \begin{bmatrix} \omega_x \\ \omega_y \\ \omega_z \end{bmatrix} \qquad (7.4.34)$$

$$\begin{cases} m_1 = \cos \alpha_1 \cdot \omega_{x1} + \cos \beta_1 \cdot m_Y + \cos \gamma_1 \cdot m_Z \\ m_2 = \cos \alpha_2 \cdot \omega_{x2} + \cos \beta_2 \cdot m_Y + \cos \gamma_2 \cdot m_Z \end{cases} \qquad (7.4.35)$$

$$\hat{\omega}_{x1} = \frac{m_1 - 0.6871 \cdot m_Y + 0.4289 \cdot m_Z}{-0.5864} \qquad (7.4.36)$$

$$\hat{\omega}_{x2} = \frac{m_2 - 0.5519 \cdot m_Y + 0.4695 \cdot m_Z}{0.6884} \qquad (7.4.37)$$

According to constrained condition (7.4.18), obtain $k_1 = 0.46, k_2 = 0.54$
The weighted integrated reconfiguration value of X-axis is

$$\hat{\omega}_x = 0.7844m_5 - 0.7844m_4 + 0.1061m_2 + 0.0318m_3$$

Table 7.3 Statistics of three-orthogonal two-inclined fault reconfiguration

Fault axis	Reconfiguration axis	Reconfiguration expressions	Error equation $D(\hat{\omega}_x)$
X	Y, Z, g_1	$\hat{\omega}_x = \frac{m_1 - 0.6871 \cdot m_Y + 0.4289 \cdot m_Z}{-0.5864}$	$74.657\sigma^2$
	Y, Z, g_2	$\hat{\omega}_x = \frac{m_2 - 0.6871 \cdot m_Y + 0.4289 \cdot m_Z}{-0.5864}$	$53.906\sigma^2$
	Y, g_1, g_2	$\hat{\omega}_x = \frac{-0.4695 \cdot m_1 + 0.0859 \cdot m_Y + 0.4289 \cdot m_2}{0.5705}$	$72.306\sigma^2$
	Z, g_1, g_2	$\hat{\omega}_x = \frac{0.5519 \cdot m_1 - 0.0859 \cdot m_Z - 0.6871 \cdot m_2}{-0.7966}$	$44.856\sigma^2$
	Y, Z, g_1, g_2	$\hat{\omega}_x = 0.7844m_2 - 0.7844m_1$ $+ 0.1061m_Y + 0.0318m_Z$	$30.615\sigma^2$
Y	X, Z, g_1	$\hat{\omega}_y = \frac{m_1 + 0.5864 \cdot m_X + 0.4289 \cdot m_Z}{0.6871}$	$54.113\sigma^2$
	X, Z, g_2	$\hat{\omega}_y = \frac{m_2 - 0.6884 \cdot m_X + 0.4695 \cdot m_Z}{0.5519}$	$84.383 \ \sigma^2$
	X, g_1, g_2	$\hat{\omega}_y = \frac{0.4695 \cdot m_1 + 0.5706 \cdot m_X - 0.4289 \cdot m_2}{0.0858}$	$4118.054\sigma^2$
	Z, g_1, g_2	$\hat{\omega}_y = \frac{0.5519 \cdot m_1 + 0.0859 \cdot m_Z - 0.6871 \cdot m_2}{-0.7966}$	$44.856\sigma^2$
	X, Z, g_1, g_2	$\hat{\omega}_y = 0.8072m_2 + 0.8070m_1$ $- 0.0825m_X + 0.7251m_Z$	$32.741\sigma^2$
Z	X, Y, g_1	$\hat{\omega}_z = \frac{m_1 + 0.5864 \cdot m_X - 0.6871 \cdot m_Y}{-0.4289}$	$140.354\sigma^2$
	X, Y, g_2	$\hat{\omega}_z = \frac{m_2 + 0.6884 \cdot m_X - 0.5519 \cdot m_Y}{-0.4695}$	$116.999\sigma^2$
	X, g_1, g_2	$\hat{\omega}_z = \frac{0.6871 \cdot m_2 - 0.7956 \cdot m_X - 0.5519 \cdot m_1}{-0.0858}$	$4118.054\sigma^2$
	Y, g_1, g_2	$\hat{\omega}_z = \frac{0.5864 \cdot m_2 - 0.7956 \cdot m_Y + 0.6884 \cdot m_1}{-0.5706}$	$72.306\sigma^2$
	X, Y, g_1, g_2	$\hat{\omega}_z = -1.1129m_2 - 1.1212m_1$ $+ 1.3400m_Y + 0.1087m_X$	$63.774\sigma^2$

The variance of reconfiguration error is

$$D(\hat{\omega}_x) = 30.615\sigma^2 \tag{7.4.38}$$

Count the fault reconfiguration results and errors of inertial devices on different main axles (Table 7.3).

From the table, we can know that when uses X, g_1, g_2 for fault reconfiguration of Y-axis and uses X, g_1, g_2 for fault reconfiguration of Z-axis, the error variance is larger, this is because under the installation of $\alpha_1 = 125.9°, \beta_1 = 46.6°, \gamma_1 = 115.4°, \alpha_2 = 46.5°, \beta_2 = 56.5°, \gamma_2 = 118°$, the physical correlation between inclined axes g_1, g_2 and Y-axis, Z-axis is small, which leads to large measurement error.

When X-axis fails, the reconfiguration error by applying the information of Y, Z, g_1, g_2 is the minimum. When Y-axis fails, the reconfiguration error by applying the information of X, Z, g_1, g_2 is the minimum. When Z-axis fails, the reconfiguration error by applying the information of X, Z, g_1, g_2 is the minimum. It means that the error variance of reconfiguration by using the information on all the remaining four axes is the minimum, with the highest accuracy of reconfiguration.

7.4.2 System-Level Fault Reconfiguration of Multi-IMUs

As far as the system-level redundant configuration of multi-IMUs, if the installation relations between the multi-sets of IMUs are calibrated, i.e., the relative installation angles between different IMUs are determined, the inertial devices in the same types on different IMUs are translated to one point. At this moment, multi-sets of IMUs could be equivalent to multi-table single set of IMU completely. The reconfiguration method may refer to Sect. 7.4.1.

Besides this, simply and practically, there are other fault reconfiguration methods for engineering. Taking the example of redundant configuration scheme of three IMUs, when one inertial device in one set of IMU fails, the whole set may be cut off, take the measurement quantity of the remaining two sets of IMUs as the output. Also only shield off the fault device on the fault IMU. The measurement quantity of other normal inertial devices in the fault IMU could be taken for output by weighting with the quantity of other two sets of IMUs. Figures 7.10 and 7.11 describe the process of fault reconfiguration of two sets of schemes respectively. The former one is simple and reliable, but with low economic efficiency and the redundancy of the system reconfiguration is decreased. The later one has complicated algorithm, but has ensured the system has certain redundant capability after the fault as much as possible, meanwhile, give consideration to economical efficiency and measurement accuracy. The scheme shall be selected comprehensively according to the characteristics and requirements of specific mission.

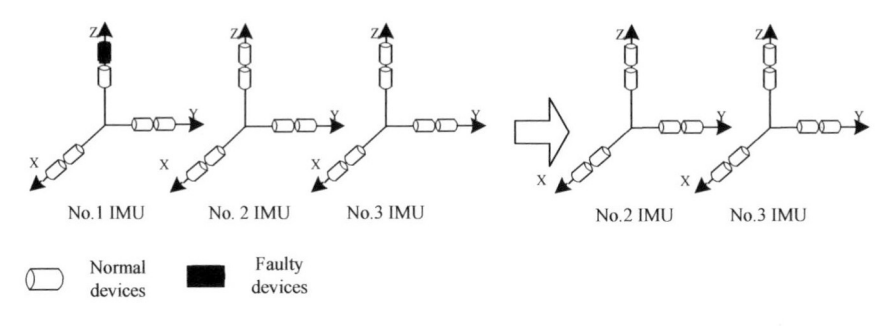

Fig. 7.10 Reconfiguration scheme of cutting off the whole IMU

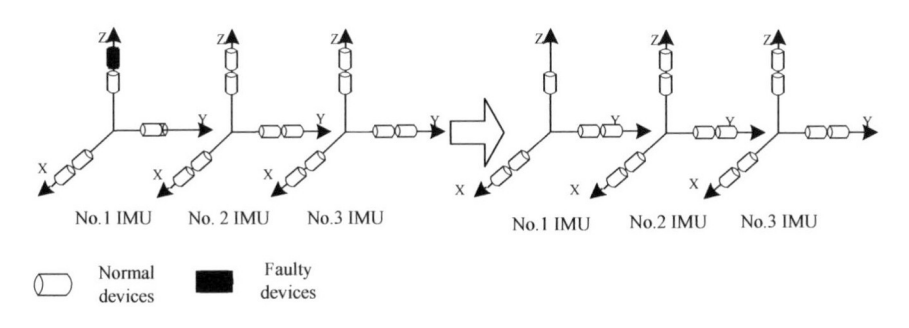

Fig. 7.11 Reconfiguration scheme of cutting off the fault inertial device

Reference Documentation

1. Li, Chaobing, Zijun Ren. 2014. Research on Configuration and Fault Reconfiguration Technology of Five Redundant Strapdown Inertial Group. *Integration of Mechanics and Electrics* 20 (2): 28–30, 78.
2. Chen, Jie, Hongyue Zhang, and Guangque Yi. 1997. Configuration Structure of Sensors and Optimization of Parity Vector in Redundancy Sensor System. *Chinese Journal of Aeronautics* 11 (3): 175–182.
3. Wang, Yinan, Kang Chen, Jie Yan. 2014. Design Method of Fault Detection Threshold of Three Strapdown Inertial Group Redundant System. *Journal of Solid Rocket Technology* 37 (4): 458–462.
4. Zhang, Lingxia, Ming Chen, and Cuiping Liu. 2005. Equivalence Between Optimal Parity Vector Method and Generalized Likelihood Ratio Test for Fault Diagnosis of Redundant Sensor. *Journal of Northwestern Polytechnical University* 23 (2): 266–270.
5. Liu, Shahong. 2012. Research on Multi-sensor Redundant Technology of Strapdown Inertial Navigation System. *Journal of Harbin Institute of Technology*.
6. Pan, Hongfei, Liqun Yuan, and Shangyun Ren. 2003. Research on Redundant Configuration of Strapdown Inertial Navigation Gyroscope. *Winged Missiles Journal* 2: 52–56.
7. Zhang, Zhixin, and Feng Zhang. 2008. Fault Detection of Strapdown Inertial Navigation System Based on Fault Tree and Singular Value Decomposition. *Journal of Chinese Inertial Technology* 16 (3): 359–363.

Chapter 8
Guidance and Midcourse Correction Technology

8.1 Introduction

The orbit of Orbital Transfer Vehicle (OTV) commonly consists of the active flight section and free flight section. Among which, the active flight section refers to the motional process of the flight vehicle under the ignition of orbit maneuver motor. The free flight section is the motional process of the flight vehicle under the actions of gravitation and various types of perturbation effects after the shutdown of orbit maneuver motor.

The orbital control of the OTV refers to the technology of orbital maneuver motor applying an external force to the centroid of flight vehicle to change its motion track. The orbit control of flight vehicle could be classified into two types, one is the orbit maneuver (or orbital transfer for simplification), i.e., the flight vehicle controls the maneuver of transfer orbit for several times and enters into nominal orbit finally with the assistance of own guidance and propulsion system. Such orbital control is commonly called guidance. Another type is the midcourse correction, i.e., to correct and control the orbit discontinuously for overcoming the perturbation to the orbit by the factors of the space environment, so as to maintain the orbit of flight vehicle to conform to the applied missions.

To save fuel and increase the carrying capacity, when the OTV enters into the nominal orbit from initial orbit, it usually maneuvers once to enter into scheduled transfer orbit for the flight vehicle to fly freely. When it moves to the terminal section of the transfer orbit, it makes another orbital transfer for the flight vehicle to enter the nominal orbit. Usually, the first type of orbital control technology will be used for designing the maneuver applied from the initial orbit to the transfer orbit and from the transfer orbit to the nominal orbit. Since the maneuver range of such two orbital transfers is larger, the sustainer motor with strong capability of orbital transfer shall be used.

Ideally, the flight vehicle may enter into nominal orbit with the orbital maneuver designed by the sustainer motor. However, during the actual flight process, due to

© Springer Nature Singapore Pte Ltd. and National Defense Industry Press, Beijing 2018
X. Li and C. Li, *Navigation and Guidance of Orbital Transfer Vehicle*, Navigation: Science and Technology, https://doi.org/10.1007/978-981-10-6334-3_8

the effects of nonspherical terrain gravitation, lunisolar attraction, atmospheric drag, sunray pressure, and the issues of injection error, navigation error, and thrust deflexion of motor existed. The actual transfer orbit of flight vehicle will inevitably deviate from the design one. To guarantee the precision of entering into the nominal orbit finally, it is essential to correct the midcourse for the actual transfer orbit. Therefore, usually, the second type of orbital control technology will be used for designing the maneuver applied, i.e., the midcourse correction. The main purpose of midcourse correction is to overcome the influence of perturbation factors and to provide better initial conditions for the first type of orbital control technology. It has a small range of maneuver. Thus, the small motor including attitude control motor shall be used. If the time of flight vehicle flying on the transfer orbit is shorter, and the influence of perturbation is within the allowable error range, the midcourse correction may be omitted.

This chapter discusses two types of orbital control of OTV, respectively. Among which, as for the first type of orbit control, it lays stress on analyzing the guidance technology, including several typical guidance methods of perturbation guidance and iterative guidance. With regard to the second type of orbital control, it emphasizes the midcourse correction technology of transfer orbit.

8.2 Guidance Technology

8.2.1 Perturbation Guidance Technology

Perturbation guidance is the guidance of the actual flight trajectory approaching to the normal trajectory, which is mainly based on Taylor expansion (perturbation theory), to realize the function of control with the perturbed shutdown equation and horizontal wizard. Commonly, the perturbed shutdown equation and horizontal wizard are called perturbation guidance. Among which, the perturbed shutdown equation is mainly realized through range control. The typically applied object of perturbation guidance is a ballistic missile. Therefore, the sample of a ballistic missile is used to describe the perturbation guidance technology. When the perturbation guidance is applied for OTV, except for the motional terms of the flight vehicle, their nature is the same.

1. **Range Control**

The flight characteristic of the active section of a ballistic missile is to fly according to the scheduled ballistic turn program setup in advance. If the flying conditions accord with the predetermined situations, under the function of program control signals, the missile will fly along the calculated normal trajectory, shut down the motor at a preset standard time, and reach to the scheduled terminal velocity and position of the active section. Thus, the missile will hit the target as long as the time control unit without error gives out the command of shutdown according to the setting time. However, actually, there are many interference factors that make the flight conditions deviate from the expected situation, resulting in launching error. The launching error includes range deviation and horizontal deviation. Commonly, range deviation is taken as the condition of the shutdown. Therefore, the function of the guidance system is to reduce the influence of interference factors through shutdown and guide, to minimize the range deviation.

Range L is the function of flight trajectory parameter $((V, r)$ and time t. Under the standard (scheduled) situations, the standard range

$$\bar{L} = l[\bar{V}_\alpha(t_k), \bar{\alpha}(t_k), \bar{t}_k] \quad \alpha = x, y, z \tag{8.2.1}$$

Here

$\bar{t}_k$ scheduled shutdown time,

$\bar{V}_\alpha(\alpha = x, y, z)$ the three components of scheduled speed in rectangular coordinate system,

$\alpha(\alpha = x, y, z)$ the three components of scheduled position shown by rectangular coordinate system,

In actual flight, due to the affections of multi-types of disturbance force and disturbance torques, the actual trajectory will deviate from the scheduled one. Hence, the actual range,

$$L = l[V_\alpha(t_k), \alpha(t_k), t_k] \quad \alpha = x, y, z \tag{8.2.2}$$

Here, the V_α, α, t_k are the actual flight speed, position, and shutdown time.

Range deviation,

$$\Delta L = L - \bar{L} \tag{8.2.3}$$

As a result of Formulas (8.2.1) and (8.2.2), the range of ballistic missile depends on the parameters of shutdown point of the active section. Taking range deviation as the shutdown control function involves seven parameters $(V_x, V_y, V_z, x, y, z, t)$. To guarantee the accuracy of range, the most direct method is to control the missile flying along the normal trajectory, i.e., the flight state that controls the terminal of the active section is fully equal to the standard value calculated in advance. However, it is very difficult for the shutdown moment to guarantee that the seven parameters are equal to the scheduled values, and it is unnecessary as well because it is possible to find one appropriate shutdown point in actual trajectory. The combined values of the seven motional parameters of such shutdown point may be equal to that of the standard shutdown point, i.e., even the flight trajectories are different, it could make $\Delta L = 0$. Figure 8.1 is the schematic diagram of different flight trajectories in the same range. Compared to the normal trajectory, the missile velocity, position, and time may not be the same, but the final range deviation shall be zero. Based on this, the indicator function of shutdown control shall be chosen as the combined value ΔL instead of the seven parameters.

Fig. 8.1 The trajectory
family entering into the same
target point

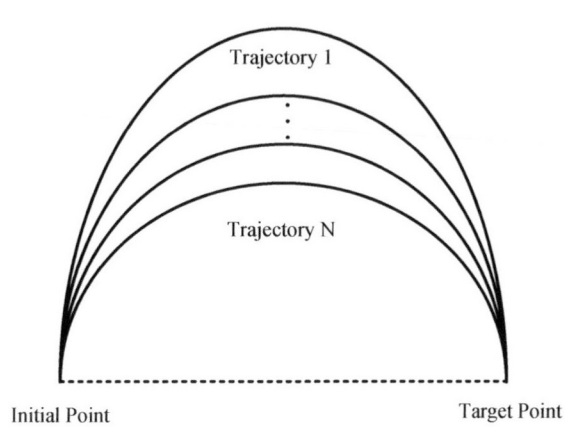

Initial Point   Target Point

Commonly, the horizontal wizard could have the minimum range deviation between the actual trajectory and normal trajectory by adjusting attitudes. The requirement of guidance calculation will be met as long as taking the first-order Taylor expansion. At this time,

$$\Delta L \triangleq J(t_k) - \bar{J}(\bar{t}_k) \tag{8.2.4}$$

Here,

$$J(t_k) = \frac{\partial L}{\partial V_x} V_x(t_k) + \frac{\partial L}{\partial V_y} V_y(t_k) + \frac{\partial L}{\partial V_z} V_z(t_k) + \frac{\partial L}{\partial x} x(t_k) + \frac{\partial L}{\partial y} y(t_k) + \frac{\partial L}{\partial z} z(t_k) + \frac{\partial L}{\partial t}(t_k)$$

$$\bar{J}(\bar{t}_k) = \frac{\partial L}{\partial V_x} \bar{V}_x(\bar{t}_k) + \frac{\partial L}{\partial V_y} \bar{V}_y(\bar{t}_k) + \frac{\partial L}{\partial V_z} \bar{V}_z(\bar{t}_k) + \frac{\partial L}{\partial x} \bar{x}(\bar{t}_k) + \frac{\partial L}{\partial y} \bar{y}(\bar{t}_k) + \frac{\partial L}{\partial z} \bar{z}(\bar{t}_k) + \frac{\partial L}{\partial t}(\bar{t}_k)$$

Formula (8.2.4) shows that even though the seven motional parameters of shutdown point are different from the standard value, as long as the combined value $J(t_k)$ is met and the standard range conditions are the same, i.e.,

$$J(t_k) = \bar{J}(\bar{t}_k) \tag{8.2.5}$$

The range deviation ΔL could be zero. Thus, $J(t)$ is defined as the shutdown characteristic quantity (also called shutdown control function), written as

$$J(t) = \sum_{i=1}^{7} K_i X_i \tag{8.2.6}$$

Here, $X_i(i = 1, 2, \ldots 7)$ shows $V_x(t), V_y(t), \ldots t$, respectively; $K_i(i = 1, 2, \ldots 7)$ shows the state variable coefficient of $\frac{\partial L}{\partial V_x}, \frac{\partial L}{\partial V_y}, \ldots, \frac{\partial L}{\partial t}$ (also called range deviation coefficient).

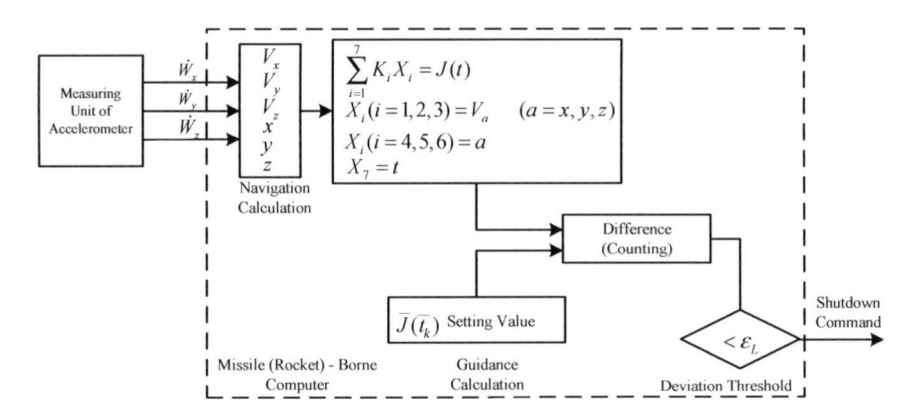

Fig. 8.2 Blocked diagram of range control of perturbation guidance system

Known from Formula (8.2.4), the perturbation guidance does not need to compare the actual state quantity and standard state quantity in real time. However, it needs to solve the state parameters near to the shutdown point and calculate the shutdown characteristic quantity according to Formula (8.2.6). Compare the actual shutdown characteristic quantity $J(t_k)$ and the setting $\bar{J}(\bar{t}_k)$ in real time, when the $J(t_k)$ and the standard shutdown characteristic quantity setup equal to or less than one permitted value ε_L, it will issue the command to shut down the motor. Thus, the amount of real-time calculation of perturbation guidance is less. Figure 8.2 is the blocked diagram of range control of perturbation guidance system.

2. Normal Steering and Lateral Steering

The purpose of normal steering is to control the flight vehicle on the radial, while lateral steering is mainly to control the flight vehicle on the shot plane (the *xoy*-plane in launching coordinate system) is shown in Fig. 8.3. By controlling the normal steering and lateral steering, the range deviation and lateral deviation could be kept at the minimum for all the time, so as to ensure the effectiveness of range shutdown control.

(1) Normal Steering

Normal steering is to control the normal direction of mass-center motion of flight vehicle in the shot plane, which mainly controls the trajectory inclination angle θ_H (the included angle between velocity vector of flight vehicle and the local level). As shown in Fig. 8.4.

As a result of Fig. 8.4, $\theta_H = \arctan\dfrac{V_z}{\sqrt{V_x^2 + V_y^2}}$, the deviation of trajectory inclination angle may be reduced via controlling the pitch angle of missile. Taking the scheduled trajectory inclination angle $\bar{\theta}_H(t)$ as the reference, and taking $\Delta\theta_H(t)$ as the normal control function, the first-order approximate expression of deviation of trajectory inclination angle at the moment of shutdown point may be written as

Fig. 8.3 Schematic diagram
of normal and lateral steering

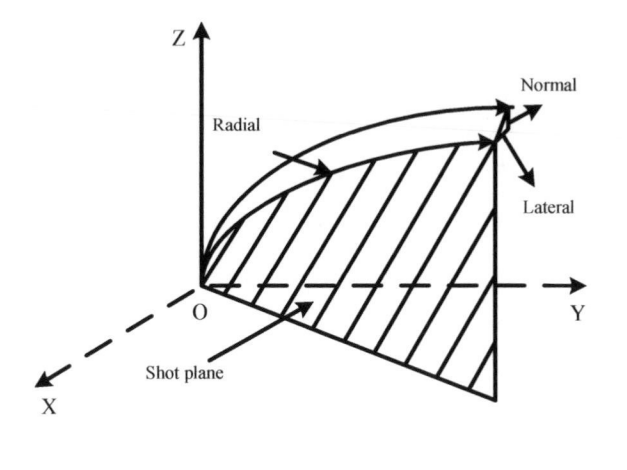

Fig. 8.4 Schematic diagram
of trajectory inclination angle

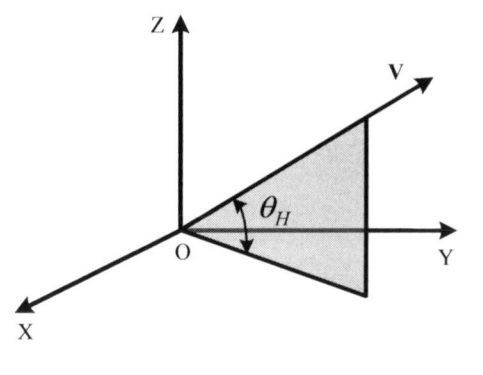

$$\Delta\theta_H(t_k) = \delta\theta_H(t_k) + \dot{\theta}_H(t_k - \bar{t}_k) \qquad (8.2.7)$$

Here, the equal time deviation

$$\delta\theta_H(t_k) = \sum E_i \delta\zeta_i \qquad (8.2.8)$$

Among them, $E_i = \left.\frac{\partial\theta_H}{\partial\zeta}\right|_{t_k}$, $\delta\zeta_i = \delta V_x, \delta V_y, \delta V_z, \delta x, \delta y, \delta z$. Range control is the first condition to achieve the goal of guidance, there exists the time $\Delta L = 0$, i.e.,

$$\Delta L = \delta L + \dot{L}(t_k - \bar{t}_k) = 0$$

Among which, $\dot{L}$ is determined by normal trajectory, thus,

$$t_k - \bar{t}_k = -\frac{\delta L}{\dot{L}} \qquad (8.2.9)$$

Put the Formulas (8.2.8) and (8.2.9) into Formula(8.2.7), there will be,

$$\Delta\theta_H(t_k) = \sum_{i=1}^{6} \left(E_i - \frac{\dot{\theta}_H}{L} a_i \right) \delta\zeta_i \tag{8.2.10}$$

Among which, the coefficient of range deviation $a_i = \frac{\partial L}{\partial V_x}, \frac{\partial L}{\partial V_y}, \cdots \frac{\partial L}{\partial V_z}\Big|_{t_k}$.

(2) Lateral Steering

Known from the previous description of range control, the shutdown adjustment could only keep the range deviation to the minimum, but the lateral deviation has not been taken into consideration. To ensure that the lateral deviation of missile falling point and that of the launch vehicle flight trajectory are less than the allowable values, lateral control shall be taken to guide the flight vehicle to fly back to the shot plane, as it is shown in Fig. 8.5.

Known from Fig. 8.5, the lateral deviation makes up one included angle $\Delta\psi$ between the actual shot plane of missile and the standard shot plane, and there is $\Delta\psi \approx \arctan\frac{\Delta H}{L}$; it is possible to control the missile heading angle to decrease the $\Delta\psi$, so as to reduce the lateral deviation.

The purpose of lateral motional control is to make the deviation of motional parameters at the shutdown moment meet the lateral deviation,

$$\Delta H(t_k) = 0 \tag{8.2.11}$$

Similar to the normal guidance mode, if it deviates beyond the first-order approximate, the lateral deviation of falling point caused by the moment of shutdown point,

$$\Delta H(t_k) = \delta H(t_k) + \dot{H}(t_k - \bar{t}_k) \tag{8.2.12}$$

Put the Formula (8.2.11) into the above-mentioned formula, and obtain,

$$\Delta H(t_k) = \delta H(t_k) - \frac{\dot{H}}{L} \delta L(t_k) = \sum_{i=1}^{6} \left(b_i - \frac{\dot{H}}{L} a_i \delta \right) \zeta_i(t_k) \tag{8.2.13}$$

Fig. 8.5 Schematic diagram of lateral deviation

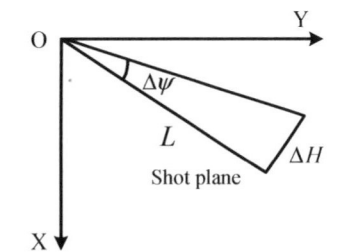

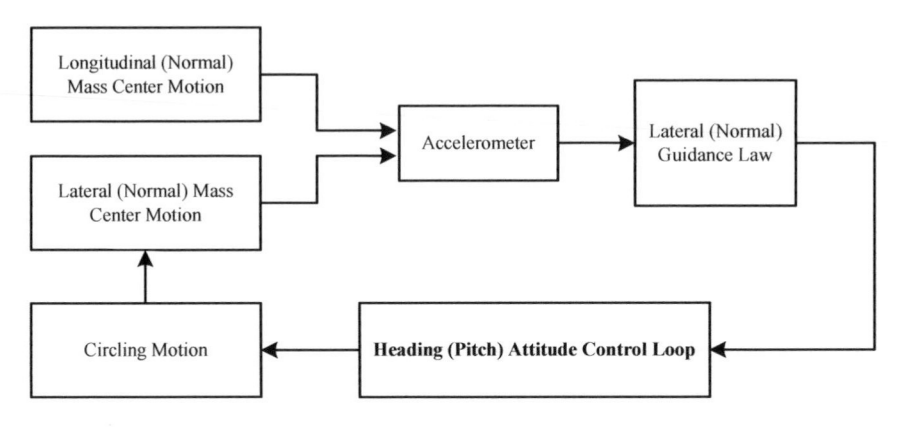

Fig. 8.6 Blocked diagram of lateral (normal) guidance system

Here, the $\dot{H}$ is determined by normal trajectory, $b_i = \frac{\partial H}{\partial V_x}, \frac{\partial H}{\partial V_y}, \frac{\partial H}{\partial V_z}, \frac{\partial H}{\partial x}, \frac{\partial H}{\partial y}, \frac{\partial H}{\partial z}\big|_{t_k}$ is the coefficient of lateral deviation.

Normal navigation is the return-to-zero control of flight vehicle deviating from the trajectory inclination angle. Lateral guidance is the return-to-zero control of flight vehicle deviating from the shot plane, these two shall control the lateral motion of the center of mass continuously, so as to form one closed loop guidance system according to the feedback control theory. The lateral (normal) guidance system calculates the lateral (normal) control functions with the information of position and velocity. Through calculating guidance, it generates the guidance signals in proportion. Such signals are sent into the yaw (pitch) channel of attitude control system continuously, to change the yaw angle (pitch angle) by the steering force of thrust vector control links, and control the motion of mass center. Since the lateral and normal guidance are to control the center of mass moving on the shot plane (in normal) and lateral plane. Commonly, they shall be analyzed according to two independent control channels. The blocked diagram of lateral (normal) guidance system is shown in Fig. 8.6.

Besides the range, the shutdown characteristic quantity, subject to the demands of the actual mission, sometimes adopts velocity and time as well. With regard to the OTV, the main purpose of the guidance is to enter into trajectory smoothly. Among the six factors that describe the major semi-axis, eccentricity, inclination angle of orbit, longitude of ascending node, argument of perigee, and true anomaly (or the time of perigee passage) of the orbit, the major semi-axis determines the operating period of orbit, which is the first premise of entry. Thus, the major semi-axis of the orbit is usually taken as the shutdown characteristic quantity, i.e., $J(t) = a(a$ is the semi-axis). At this moment, the corresponding normal guidance is mainly pertinent to the eccentricity. It could be fulfilled by controlling the inclination angle of local horizontal velocity, while the lateral guidance is mainly pertinent to the tilt angle of the orbit.

8.2.2 *Iterative Guidance Technology*

Theoretically, the guidance of flight vehicle is the optimal control problem that takes the motion of center of mass as the state equation, the instantaneous state as the initial value, the target state as the terminal constraint, the thrust direction as the control vector, and the minimum flight time as the performance index. With the optimal control theory, one group of extremal conditions, state equation, adjoint equation, and transversality condition that take thrust direction as the control variables could be derived. The solutions of such group of equations may obtain the expressions (guidance equation) and corresponding optimal orbit of the optimal control direction vector. However, in actual applications, the guidance computer carried by the flight vehicle could not calculate the complicated solution procedure of the above-mentioned equations. Therefore, it needs to simplify the equation set to certain extent so as to obtain the equations that fit for the solution of guidance computer. Iterative guidance is one of the simplification technologies. The solution of the optimal injection point and optimal trajectory continuously through iteration is called iterative guidance.

1. Flight Vehicle Equation of Motion

Set up the equation of motion in the orbital coordinate system of injection point. The subscript of the quantity related to the orbital coordinate system of injection point is shown by *ocf*. Considering the flight vehicle is basically at vacuum environment in actual flight, without taking the atmospheric influence, the control system may guarantee that the rolling angle is approximate aero, and in deriving iterative guidance, assumed flat Earth, after being simplified, the mass-center dynamics of the injection point of the flight vehicle is obtained as follows:

$$\begin{bmatrix} \ddot{X}_{ocf} \\ \ddot{Y}_{ocf} \\ \ddot{Z}_{ocf} \end{bmatrix} = \frac{F}{m} \begin{bmatrix} \cos \varphi_{ocf} \cos \psi_{ocf} \\ \sin \varphi_{ocf} \cos \psi_{ocf} \\ -\sin \psi_{ocf} \end{bmatrix} + \begin{bmatrix} g_{ocf\,x} \\ g_{ocf\,y} \\ g_{ocf\,z} \end{bmatrix} \tag{8.2.14}$$

Among which, $\begin{bmatrix} X & Y & Z \end{bmatrix}^{\mathrm{T}}$ is the position vector of flight vehicle, F is the thrust of flight vehicle, m is the mass of the flight vehicle, φ is the pitch angle, ψ is the yawing angle, and g is the gravitational acceleration.

Assuming the local planarization of the track between the instantaneous point and the injection point of the flight vehicle, the gravitational acceleration vector is approximately the average value between the gravitational acceleration vector of instantaneous point and that of the injection point, that will be,

$$\begin{bmatrix} g_{ocf\,x} \\ g_{ocf\,y} \\ g_{ocf\,z} \end{bmatrix} = \frac{1}{2} \left(\begin{bmatrix} g_{ocf0\,x} \\ g_{ocf0\,y} \\ g_{ocf0\,z} \end{bmatrix} + \begin{bmatrix} g_{ocff\,x} \\ g_{ocff\,y} \\ g_{ocff\,z} \end{bmatrix} \right) \tag{8.2.15}$$

Here, $g_{ocf\,x}$, $g_{ocf\,y}$, and $g_{ocf\,z}$ are the three components of the average gravitational acceleration in the injection point orbital system. The g_{ocf0x}, g_{ocf0y}, and g_{ocf0z} are the three components of the gravitational acceleration at the instantaneous point of the flight vehicle in the orbital system at the injection point; the $g_{ocff\,x}$, $g_{ocff\,y}$, and $g_{ocff\,z}$ are the three components of the gravitational acceleration of injection point of the flight vehicle in the orbital system of the injection point.

The mass-center dynamic equation of flight vehicle,

$$\begin{bmatrix} \dot{X}_{ocf} \\ \dot{Y}_{ocf} \\ \dot{Z}_{ocf} \end{bmatrix} = \begin{bmatrix} V_{xocf} \\ V_{yocf} \\ V_{zocf} \end{bmatrix} \tag{8.2.16}$$

Among which, $\begin{bmatrix} V_x & V_y & V_z \end{bmatrix}^{\mathrm{T}}$ is the velocity vector of flight vehicle.

2. Description of Optimal Control Problem

Since the thrust of flight vehicle motor is constant, the $F = \text{const}$ in Eq. (8.2.14). Also known $F = \dot{m}Vex$, in it, $\dot{m}$ is the second consumption, Vex is specific thrust. As for most of the flight vehicle orbital missions, the minimum fuel consumption is expected during the process of injection, i.e., the effective mass of injection is the maximum. Since $\dot{m}$ is one constant, the performance index is equivalent to the minimum time, namely,

$$J = \int_0^t \mathrm{d}t \tag{8.2.17}$$

Following is the state equation of determining optimal control problem. Write Eqs. (8.2.14) and (8.2.16) in the form of state space, the state variables are as follows: $X = \begin{bmatrix} \dot{X}_{ocf} & X_{ocf} & \dot{Y}_{ocf} & Y_{ocf} & \dot{Z}_{ocf} & Z_{ocf} \end{bmatrix}^{\mathrm{T}}$, and obtain,

$$\dot{X} = AX + Bu + C \tag{8.2.18}$$

In it

$$A = \begin{bmatrix} 0 & 0 & 0 & 0 & 0 & 0 \\ 1 & 0 & 0 & 0 & 0 & 0 \\ 0 & 0 & 0 & 0 & 0 & 0 \\ 0 & 0 & 1 & 0 & 0 & 0 \\ 0 & 0 & 0 & 0 & 0 & 0 \\ 0 & 0 & 0 & 0 & 1 & 0 \end{bmatrix}, B = \frac{F}{m}, u = \begin{bmatrix} \cos \varphi_{ocf} \cos \psi_{ocf} \\ 0 \\ \sin \varphi_{ocf} \cos \psi_{ocf} \\ 0 \\ -\sin \psi_{ocf} \\ 0 \end{bmatrix}, C = \begin{bmatrix} g_{ocf\,x} \\ 0 \\ g_{ocf\,y} \\ 0 \\ g_{ocf\,z} \\ 0 \end{bmatrix}.$$

Since X is the state variable, the initial value and final value shall be determined. From the states (velocity, position) of the flight vehicle at the present moment and injection, the X initial value of $X_i = \begin{bmatrix} \dot{X}_{ocfi} & X_{ocfi} & \dot{Y}_{ocfi} & Y_{ocfi} & \dot{Z}_{ocfi} & Z_{ocfi} \end{bmatrix}^{\mathrm{T}}$, and the X final value of $X_f = \begin{bmatrix} \dot{X}_{ocff} & X_{ocff} & \dot{Y}_{ocff} & Y_{ocff} & \dot{Z}_{ocff} & Z_{ocff} \end{bmatrix}^{\mathrm{T}}$, u is the control variable.

Equations (8.2.17) and (8.2.18) form one optimal control problem. The solution of the optimal control problem is to solve the change rule of u, to transfer the whole system from the initial state to the final state in the minimum time. When it obtains the change rule of u, the instruction of flying attitude of the flight vehicle could be known.

3. To Solve the Optimal Control Problem

To solve the above-mentioned optimal control problem, write the Hamiltonian function.

$$H = \lambda_1 \left(\frac{F}{m} \cos \varphi_{ocf} \cos \psi_{ocf} + g_{ocf\,x} \right) + \lambda_2 X_{ocf} + \lambda_3 \left(\frac{F}{m} \sin \varphi_{ocf} \cos \psi_{ocf} + g_{ocf\,y} \right)$$
$$+ \lambda_4 Y_{ocf} + \lambda_5 \left(-\frac{F}{m} \sin \psi_{ocf} + g_{ocf\,z} \right) + \lambda_6 + 1$$

$$(8.2.19)$$

From the extremal conditions of optimal control, we could obtain,

$$\frac{\partial H}{\partial u} = 0 \qquad\qquad (8.2.20)$$

That is

$$\begin{bmatrix} \lambda_1 \sin \varphi_{ocf} \cos \psi_{ocf} - \lambda_3 \cos \varphi_{ocf} \cos \psi_{ocf} \\ \lambda_1 \cos \varphi_{ocf} \sin \psi_{ocf} + \lambda_3 \sin \varphi_{ocf} \sin \psi_{ocf} + \lambda_5 \cos \psi_{ocf} \end{bmatrix} = 0 \qquad (8.2.21)$$

The adjoint equation is

$$\dot{\lambda} = -\frac{\partial H}{\partial X} \qquad\qquad (8.2.22)$$

That is

$$\begin{bmatrix} \dot{\lambda}_1 \\ \dot{\lambda}_2 \\ \dot{\lambda}_3 \\ \dot{\lambda}_4 \\ \dot{\lambda}_5 \\ \dot{\lambda}_6 \end{bmatrix} = \begin{bmatrix} -\lambda_2 \\ 0 \\ -\lambda_4 \\ 0 \\ -\lambda_6 \\ 0 \end{bmatrix} \qquad\qquad (8.2.23)$$

The transversality condition is

$$\lambda \delta X \big|_{t_f} = 0 \qquad\qquad (8.2.24)$$

That is

$$
\begin{bmatrix}
\lambda_1 \delta X_1 \\
\lambda_2 \delta X_2 \\
\lambda_3 \delta X_3 \\
\lambda_4 \delta X_4 \\
\lambda_5 \delta X_5 \\
\lambda_6 \delta X_6
\end{bmatrix} = 0
\tag{8.2.25}
$$

To integrate Eq. (8.2.23), obtain,

$$
\begin{cases}
\lambda_1 = \lambda_{10} - \lambda_{20} t \\
\lambda_3 = \lambda_{30} - \lambda_{40} t \\
\lambda_5 = \lambda_{50} - \lambda_{60} t
\end{cases}
\tag{8.2.26}
$$

Here, the $\lambda_{10}, \lambda_{20} \ldots \lambda_{60}$ are the constants of integration.

To determine the velocity components of the target point $\left(\dot{X}_{ocff}, \dot{Y}_{ocff}, \dot{Z}_{ocff}\right)$ and the position $\left(Y_{ocff}, Z_{ocff}\right)$, if the X_{ocff} is uncertain, there is

$$
\lambda_{20} = 0
$$

$$
\begin{cases}
\lambda_1 = \lambda_{10} \\
\lambda_3 = \lambda_{30} - \lambda_{40} t \\
\lambda_5 = \lambda_{50} - \lambda_{60} t
\end{cases}
\tag{8.2.27}
$$

Solve Eqs. (8.2.21) and (8.2.27), and gain

$$
\begin{cases}
\tan \varphi_{ocf} = \frac{\lambda_{30} - \lambda_{40} t}{\lambda_{10}} \\
\tan \psi_{ocf} = \frac{\lambda_{50} - \lambda_{60} t}{\lambda_{10} \cos \varphi_{ocf} + (\lambda_{30} - \lambda_{40} t) \sin \varphi_{ocf}}
\end{cases}
\tag{8.2.28}
$$

The expression of control angle relies on the determination of constant of integration λ_{i0}. Since the solution of the above-mentioned equation is very complicated, under the assumption of constant thrust, constant specific thrust, and homogenous gravity field, the following formula is usually used for giving the approximate analytical form of the optimal control angle in the iterative guidance,

$$
\begin{cases}
\varphi_{ocf} = \bar{\varphi}_{ocf} - K_{\varphi 1} + K_{\varphi 2} t \\
\psi_{ocf} = \bar{\psi}_{ocf} - K_{\psi 1} + K_{\psi 2} t
\end{cases}
\tag{8.2.29}
$$

Here, the $\bar{\varphi}_{ocf}$ and $\bar{\psi}_{ocf}$ adopt the optimal control principle to control the attitude angle that saves the most fuel as long as meeting the terminal velocity constraint, such quantity is the main part of the whole control attitude angle. The control quantity that meets the position constraint of injection point is the secondary part of the instruction of the attitude angle, the $K_{\varphi 1}$, $K_{\varphi 2}$, $K_{\psi 1}$, and $K_{\psi 2}$ are the parameters of the additional small angle of the radius vector of the injection point. Therefore, the core of the iterative guidance is to solve the above-mentioned six parameters.

The solution of the iterative guidance parameters consists of two parts, i.e., prediction and correction. The prediction quantity includes the remaining flight time, the predicted value of the geocentric angle of instantaneous injection point related to the remaining time, thrust integration, gravitational integration, position, and velocity of the injection point. Correction refers to the process of solving optimal control solution with the prediction quantity and expected quantity. The process of correction is the general summary of the steps.

Remaining time refers to the time of the flight vehicle from the concurrent point to the shutdown point (the injection point). The geocentric angle is the angle of the injection angle corresponding to the concurrent moment, which is used for calculating the coordinate transfer matrix A_{icf}^{ocf}. The thrust integration refers to the increments of velocity and position of flight vehicle produced by thrust during the entire flight process. The former one is called the first integral of thrust, and the latter is called the double integral of thrust. The thrust integration refers to the increment of velocity and position that is only produced by gravitational force during the entire flight process. The former one is called the first integral of thrust and the latter is called the double integral of thrust.

4. Prediction Process

The process of prediction contains the solution of remaining time, solution of geocentric angle, and calculation of thrust integration and gravitational integration.

a. Calculate remaining time

Use the Ziolkovsky Formula to give one prediction formula of the remaining time. It assumes the instantaneous guidance moment of the flight vehicle is 0, the mass is m_0, shutdown time is t_s, the remaining time is $t_g = t_s - 0 = t_s$, and velocity increment is ΔV, and obtains the formula,

$$t_g = t_h \left(1 - e^{\frac{\Delta V}{I_{sp}}} \right) \tag{8.2.30}$$

Among which, $t_h = \frac{m_0}{\dot{m}}$, $\dot{m} = \frac{F}{I_{sp}}$ is the second consumption, I_{sp} is the specific thrust.

Because the concurrent moment of flight vehicle could not obtain ΔV, the ΔV is one prediction quantity. Therefore, to solve the t_g, it needs one iterative process. It assumes V_{xocff}, V_{yocff}, and V_{zocff} are the velocity components of the injection point in the orbital coordinate system of the injection point, the V_{xocf0}, V_{yocf0}, and V_{zocf0} are the velocity components of the instantaneous moment of the flight vehicle in the orbital coordinate system of the injection point, thus,

$$\Delta V = \sqrt{\left(V_{xocf} - V_{xocf0} - g_{xocf}t_g\right)^2 + \left(V_{yocf} - V_{yocf0} - g_{yocf}t_g\right)^2 + \left(V_{zocf} - V_{zocf0} - g_{zocf}t_g\right)^2}$$

$$(8.2.31)$$

Formulas (8.2.32) and (8.2.33) form the iterative process of predicting the remaining time t_g

b. Calculate Thrust Integration

Assuming the thurst as one constant, the analytical results of thrust integration could be drawn out. The component of the thrust term in the orbital coordinate system of the injection point is $\frac{F}{m}\begin{bmatrix} \cos\varphi_{ocf}\cos\psi_{ocf} \\ \sin\varphi_{ocf}\cos\psi_{ocf} \\ -\sin\psi_{ocf} \end{bmatrix}$. Assuming the remaining flight time has been obtained, the first integral of thrust is

$$V_{\text{thrust}} = \begin{bmatrix} \int_0^{t_g} \frac{F}{m}\cos\varphi_{ocf}\cos\psi_{ocf}dt \\ \int_0^{t_g} \frac{F}{m}\sin\varphi_{ocf}\cos\psi_{ocf}dt \\ -\int_0^{t_g} \frac{F}{m}\sin\psi_{ocf}dt \end{bmatrix} \qquad (8.2.32)$$

The double integral of thrust is

$$R_{\text{thrust}} = \begin{bmatrix} \int_0^{t_g}\int_0^{s} \frac{F}{m}\cos\varphi_{ocf}\cos\psi_{ocf}dsdt \\ \int_0^{t_g}\int_0^{s} \frac{F}{m}\sin\varphi_{ocf}\cos\psi_{ocf}dsdt \\ -\int_0^{t_g}\int_0^{s} \frac{F}{m}\sin\psi_{ocf}dsdt \end{bmatrix} \qquad (8.2.33)$$

Put the Formulas (8.2.29) and $\frac{F}{m} = \frac{I_{sp}}{t_h - t}$ into Formula (8.2.32), and considering every instantaneous flight moment of the flight vehicle because the $\bar{\varphi}_{ocf}$ and $\bar{\psi}_{ocf}$ are the constant vectors of the concurrent moment that meet the velocity vector of the injection point during the process of integration, and it shall be taken as one constant. Since the regulated quantity of position vector $-K_{\varphi1} + K_{\varphi2}t$ and $-K_{\psi1} + K_{\psi2}t$ are small, they shall be taken as the small quantity during the process of integration. In addition, in preliminary design of trajectory for most of the flight vehicles, the yaw angles are designed to be 0, thus, $\psi_{ocf} \approx 0$. And since the above-mentioned $-K_{\varphi1} + K_{\varphi2}t$ and $-K_{\psi1} + K_{\psi2}t$ are small, following functions are defined,

$$F_0(t) = \int_0^t \frac{I_{sp}}{t_h - t}dt = I_{sp}\ln\frac{t_h}{t_h - t} \qquad (8.2.34)$$

$$F_1(t) = \int_0^t \frac{I_{sp}}{t_h - t} t\,dt = t_h F_0(t) - I_{sp} \cdot t \qquad (8.2.35)$$

Omitting the second-order small, Formula (8.2.32) may derive and obtain,

$$\boldsymbol{V}_{thrust} = \begin{bmatrix} F_0(t_g)\cos(\bar{\varphi}_{ocf})\cos(\bar{\psi}_{ocf}) + F_0(t_g)K_{\varphi 1}\sin(\bar{\varphi}_{ocf})\cos(\bar{\psi}_{ocf}) \\ -F_1(t_g)K_{\varphi 2}\sin(\bar{\varphi}_{ocf})\cos(\bar{\psi}_{ocf}) \\ F_0(t_g)\sin(\bar{\varphi}_{ocf})\cos(\bar{\psi}_{ocf}) + F_0(t_g)K_{\varphi 1}\cos(\bar{\varphi}_{ocf})\cos(\bar{\psi}_{ocf}) \\ -F_1(t_g)K_{\varphi 2}\cos(\bar{\varphi}_{ocf})\cos(\bar{\psi}_{ocf}) \\ F_0(t_g)K_{\psi 1}\cos(\bar{\psi}_{ocf}) - F_1(t_g)K_{\psi 2}\cos(\bar{\psi}_{ocf}) \end{bmatrix} \qquad (8.2.36)$$

That is the formula of the first integration of thrust.

Similarly, as for double integral of thrust, following functions are defined,

$$F_2(t) = \int_0^t \int_0^s \frac{I_{sp}}{t_h - t} dt\,ds = F_0(t) \cdot t - F_1(t) \qquad (8.2.37)$$

$$F_3(t) = \int_0^t \int_0^s \frac{I_{sp}}{t_h - t} t\,dt\,ds = F_2(t) \cdot t_h - \frac{t^2 I_{sp}}{2} \qquad (8.2.38)$$

Obtains,

$$\boldsymbol{R}_{thrust} = \begin{bmatrix} F_2(t_g)\cos(\bar{\varphi}_{ocf})\cos(\bar{\psi}_{ocf}) + F_2(t_g)K_{\varphi 1}\sin(\bar{\varphi}_{ocf})\cos(\bar{\psi}_{ocf}) \\ -F_3(t_g)K_{\varphi 2}\sin(\bar{\varphi}_{ocf})\cos(\bar{\psi}_{ocf}) \\ F_2(t_g)\sin(\bar{\varphi}_{ocf})\cos(\bar{\psi}_{ocf}) + F_2(t_g)K_{\varphi 1}\cos(\bar{\varphi}_{ocf})\cos(\bar{\psi}_{ocf}) \\ -F_3(t_g)K_{\varphi 2}\cos(\bar{\varphi}_{ocf})\cos(\bar{\psi}_{ocf}) \\ F_2(t_g)K_{\psi 1}\cos(\bar{\psi}_{ocf}) - F_3(t_g)K_{\psi 2}\cos(\bar{\psi}_{ocf}) \end{bmatrix}$$

$$(8.2.39)$$

That is the formula of double integral of thrust.

c. Calculate the Gravitational Integration

The calculation of gravitational integration is similar to that of thrust integration, the analytic method or numerical integration may be used. When it obtains the simplified form of the optimal control solution, we could calculate the analytic method, and may also calculate with the method of numerical integration. This is the analytical forms of gravitational integration.

From the constant gravitational force model, at every instantaneous moment of flight vehicle flying, the gravitational acceleration is constant, the first integral of gravitational force could be obtained as follows:

$$V_{\text{gravity}} = \begin{bmatrix} g_{xocf} t_g \\ g_{yocf} t_g \\ g_{zocf} t_g \end{bmatrix} \tag{8.2.40}$$

The double integral of gravitational force is

$$R_{\text{gravity}} = \begin{bmatrix} \frac{1}{2} g_{xocf} t_g^2 \\ \frac{1}{2} g_{yocf} t_g^2 \\ \frac{1}{2} g_{zocf} t_g^2 \end{bmatrix} \tag{8.2.41}$$

d. Calculate by taking geocentric angle as the terminal conditions,

Visually, as for the established flight mission, the velocity and position of the injection point are fixed; however, with regard to iterative guidance, it could only guarantee the three velocity vectors V_{xocff}, V_{yocff}, and V_{zocff} and two position vectors Y_{ocff} and Z_{ocff} of the injection point in the orbital coordinate system. The iterative guidance could only meet five components to the maximum. For the flight missions of most of the launch vehicles, to meet the major semi-axis, eccentricity, and inclination angle of orbit, the longitude of ascending node is the main data. Following it, convert the constraints of the orbital elements of injection points into the velocity and coordinate constraint of guidance coordinate system, and draw out the conclusion as follow:

(1) To meet the tilt angle of orbit i, the longitude of ascending node Ω, it needs to guarantee $Z_{ocff} = 0$, $V_{zocff} = 0$. Among which, Z_{ocff} is the radius vector component in Z-direction of the injection point in orbital coordinate system. V_{zocff} is the velocity component of injection point in Z-direction in orbital coordinate system.

(2) If it meets Condition (1) $Z_{ocff} = 0$, $V_{zocff} = 0$, and another condition $X_{ocff} = 0$, the major semi-axis a, eccentricity e, and the true anomaly f have the relations as follows:

$$Y_{ocff} = \frac{a(1 - e^2)}{1 + e \cos f}$$

$$V_{xocff} = \frac{\sqrt{\mu/a(1 - e^2)}}{Y_{ocff}} \tag{8.2.42}$$

$$V_{yocff} = e \sin f \sqrt{\frac{\mu}{a(1 - e^2)}}$$

Thus, when $Z_{ocff} = 0$, $V_{zocff} = 0$, and $X_{ocff} = 0$, the three components of Y_{ocff}, V_{xocff}, and V_{yocff} may ensure the major semi-axis a, eccentricity e, and the true anomaly f. However, during actual process it is difficult to meet the condition of $X_{ocff} = 0$; therefore, it is an assumption. When it meets the three velocity components of V_{xocff}, V_{yocff}, and V_{zocff} as well as the two position components of Y_{ocff} and Z_{ocff}, the X_{ocff} will be met as possible. Since the position vector X_{ocff} has not been assured, the geocentric angle could be taken as one variable quantity, also may be one constant. When the geocentric angle is taken as one variable quantity, it shall be predicted in calculating guidance. Following is the process of predicting the geocentric angle.

The geocentric angle consists of two parts, one is the geocentric angle ϕ_i of the projection of the instantaneous moment of the flight vehicle on the injection orbital plane, the other part is the included angle between the radius vector of projection point for the flight vehicle instantaneous moment and the estimated radius vector ϕ_p of the position of the injection point.

To solve the ϕ_i, the formula of calculating ϕ_i in the orbital coordinate system (turns the coordinate system to geocentric angle $(\omega + f)$ along the Z-axis) of the ascending node, i.e., to turn to the orbital coordinate system of the injection point)

$$\phi_i = \tan^{-1}\left(\frac{x_{Rcf}}{y_{Rcf}}\right) \tag{8.2.43}$$

Among which, the x_{Rcf} and y_{Rcf} are the position components of flight vehicle instantaneous moment on X-axis and Y-axis in orbital coordinate system of the ascending node.

The transfer relations from launching inertial system to orbital coordinate system of ascending node is

$$M_1 = M_y(i) \bullet M_z(-\Delta\Omega) \bullet M_y(-90°) \bullet M_z(B_0) \bullet M_y(A_0) \tag{8.2.44}$$

Considering the origin is the Earth's core, other axle are the coordinate system S_1 that is parallel with the launching inertial system, its subscript is shown by fag. Assuming the position vector of instantaneous moment of flight vehicle in S_1 system is $r_{fag} = [x_{fag}, y_{fag}, z_{fag}]^T$, the velocity vector is $v_{fag} = [v_{xfag}, v_{yfag}, v_{zfag}]^T$, in every cycle of guidance calculation, the r_{fag} and v_{fag} are given. Assuming the position component of aerocraft instantaneous moment in Z-axis of orbital coordinate system of ascending node is z_{Rcf}, the velocity in orbital coordinate system of ascending node is $v_{Rcf} = [v_{xRcf}, v_{yRcf}, v_{zRcf}]^T$, then,

$$\begin{bmatrix} x_{Rcf} \\ y_{Rcf} \\ z_{Rcf} \end{bmatrix} = M_1 \begin{bmatrix} x_{fag} \\ y_{fag} \\ z_{fag} \end{bmatrix} \tag{8.2.45}$$

$$
\begin{bmatrix} v_{xRcf} \\ v_{yRcf} \\ v_{zRcf} \end{bmatrix} = \boldsymbol{M}_1 \begin{bmatrix} v_{xfag} \\ v_{yfag} \\ v_{zfag} \end{bmatrix}
\tag{8.2.46}
$$

ϕ_p may be calculated approximately by the component of the projection of the flight vehicle instantaneous velocity vector on the local level as the initial velocity, the projection of the acceleration vector produced by the thrust of the sustainer motor on the flight course of the acceleration of local level component. As the flight vehicle approaches toward the target point, the authenticity which is represented increases. Specifically, assuming the pitch angle and yaw angle of flight vehicle in launching inertial system as φ_{fag} and ψ_{fag}, respectively, the acceleration produced by the sustainer motor in launching inertial system is

$$
\boldsymbol{a}_{fag} = \frac{F}{m} \begin{bmatrix} \cos \varphi_{fag} \cos \psi_{fag} \\ \sin \varphi_{fag} \cos \psi_{fag} \\ -\sin \psi_{fag} \end{bmatrix}
\tag{8.2.47}
$$

The acceleration produced by sustainer motor in orbital coordinate system of ascending node is

$$
\boldsymbol{a}_{Rcf} = \boldsymbol{M}_1 \boldsymbol{a}_{fag}
\tag{8.2.48}
$$

Assuming the components of $\boldsymbol{a}_{Rcf}$ in X-axis and Y-axis as a_{xRcf} and a_{yRcf}, respectively, the depletion time within the orbital plane is

$$
t_{hxy} = \frac{I_{sp}}{\sqrt{a_{xRcf}^2 + a_{yRcf}^2}}
\tag{8.2.49}
$$

Similar to the process of previously calculated thrust integration, functions defined are as follows:

$$
F_0(t)_{Rcf} = \int_0^t \frac{I_{sp}}{t_{hxy} - t} \mathrm{d}t = I_{sp} \ln \frac{t_{hxy}}{t_{hxy} - t}
\tag{8.2.50}
$$

$$
F_1(t)_{Rcf} = \int_0^t \frac{I_{sp}}{t_{hxy} - t} t \mathrm{d}t = t_{hxy} F_0(t)_{Rcf} - I_{sp} \cdot t
\tag{8.2.51}
$$

$$
F_2(t)_{Rcf} = \int_0^t \int_0^s \frac{I_{sp}}{t_{hxy} - t} \mathrm{d}t \mathrm{d}s = F_0(t)_{Rcf} \cdot t - F_1(t)_{Rcf}
\tag{8.2.52}
$$

Assuming θ_i and θ_f as the ballistic tilt angles of flight vehicle at the instantaneous moment and injection moment corresponding to local level. As for injection, $V_{xyRcf}t_g \cos\theta_i + F_2(t_g)_{Rcf} \cos\theta_f$ may be used to approximately calculate the flight range of flight vehicle on the orbital plane of injection (conversely, if from high orbit to low orbit, the function of speed reduction of sustainer motor may be approximated to the flight range by $V_{xyRcf}t_g \cos\theta_i - F_2(t_g)_{Rcf} \cos\theta_f$). Among which,

$$V_{xyRcf} = \sqrt{v_{xRcf}^2 + v_{yRcf}^2}, \cos\theta_i = \frac{\left| x_{Rcf} v_{yRcf} - y_{Rcf} v_{xRcf} \right|}{V_{xyRcf}\sqrt{x_{Rcf}^2 + y_{yRcf}^2}}.$$

θ_f is in connection with the terminal constraint. After constrains, the position and velocity vectors of target point in orbital coordinate system of assigned injection point, the position and velocity of orbital coordinate system of ascending node transferred are, respectively, $r_{Rcff} = [x_{Rcff}, y_{Rcff}, z_{Rcff}]^T$ and $v_{Rcff} = [v_{xRcff}, v_{yRcff}, v_{zRcff}]^T$, then $\cos\theta_f = \frac{\left| x_{Rcff} v_{yRcff} - y_{Rcff} v_{xRcff} \right|}{V_{xyRcff}\sqrt{x_{Rcff}^2 + y_{yRcff}^2}}.$

Among which, $V_{xyRcff} = \sqrt{v_{xRcff}^2 + v_{yRcff}^2}.$

After it calculates the flight range of flight vehicle on orbital plane of injection, since the volume of Y-axis component y_{ocff} of the constrained vector of terminal position in orbital coordinate system of the injection point is far more larger than the flight range, the ϕ_p calculating formula is

$$\phi_p = \tan^{-1}\left(\frac{V_{xyRcf}t_g \cos\theta_i - F_2(t_g)_{Rcf} \cos\theta_f}{y_{ocff}} \right) \approx \frac{V_{xyRcf}t_g \cos\theta_i - F_2(t_g)_{Rcf} \cos\theta_f}{y_{ocff}}$$

$$(8.2.53)$$

5. Correction Process

On the basis of obtaining the prediction quantity, set up constraint equation and solve the parameters $\bar{\varphi}_{ocf}$, $\bar{\psi}_{ocf}$, $K_{\varphi 1}$, $K_{\varphi 2}$, $K_{\psi 1}$, and $K_{\psi 2}$ of guidance equation.

First of all, only in the situation of velocity constraint, the velocity increment needed is

$$\Delta V = V_{ocff} - V_{ocf0} - V_{gravity} \qquad (8.2.54)$$

Among which, the V_{ocff} is the speed of injection point, i.e., the expected orbital velocity. V_{ocf0} is the velocity vector of the flight vehicle at concurrent moment. Such velocity gain is provided by thrust. It is not difficult to understand that if the thrust direction of flight vehicle motor is the same as the ΔV then it could meet the velocity gain to the greatest extent. Obtain from the geometrical relationship,

$$\begin{cases} \bar{\varphi}_{ocf} = \tan^{-1}\left(\dfrac{V_{yocff}-V_{yocf0}-g_{yocf}t_g}{V_{xocff}-V_{xocf0}-g_{xocf}t_g}\right) \\ \bar{\psi}_{ocf} = -\sin^{-1}\left(\dfrac{V_{zocff}-V_{zocf0}-g_{zocf}t_g}{\Delta V}\right) \end{cases} \tag{8.2.55}$$

Furthermore, $-K_{\varphi 1}+K_{\varphi 2}t$ and $-K_{\psi 1}+K_{\psi 2}t$ are the vector direction of injection to ensure the upper stage of the flight vehicle. If the form of control angle removes the affections of $-K_{\varphi 1}+K_{\varphi 2}t$, $-K_{\psi 1}+K_{\psi 2}t$, then,

$$\begin{cases} \varphi_{ocf} = \bar{\varphi}_{ocf} \\ \psi_{ocf} = \bar{\psi}_{ocf} \end{cases} \tag{8.2.56}$$

Put the above formula into Formula (8.2.32), similar to the previous calculation process, and obtain,

$$\boldsymbol{V}_{\text{thrust}}\left(\bar{\varphi}_{ocf},\bar{\psi}_{ocf}\right) = \begin{bmatrix} F0(t_g)\cos\left(\bar{\varphi}_{ocf}\right)\cos\left(\bar{\psi}_{ocf}\right) \\ F0(t_g)\sin\left(\bar{\varphi}_{ocf}\right)\cos\left(\bar{\psi}_{ocf}\right) \\ 0 \end{bmatrix} \tag{8.2.57}$$

The form of gravitational integration has not changed,

$$\boldsymbol{V}_{\text{gravity}}\left(\bar{\varphi}_{ocf},\bar{\psi}_{ocf}\right) = \begin{bmatrix} g_{xocf}t_g \\ g_{yocf}t_g \\ g_{zocf}t_g \end{bmatrix} \tag{8.2.58}$$

Firstly, calculate the terminal velocity $\boldsymbol{V}_{ocff}$ with the Formula (8.2.56) only, and set up the formula as follows:

$$\boldsymbol{V}_{ocff}\left(\bar{\varphi}_{ocf},\bar{\psi}_{ocf}\right) = \boldsymbol{V}_{\text{thrust}}\left(\bar{\varphi}_{ocf},\bar{\psi}_{ocf}\right) + \boldsymbol{V}_{\text{gravity}}\left(\bar{\varphi}_{ocf},\bar{\psi}_{ocf}\right) + \boldsymbol{V}_{ocf0} \tag{8.2.59}$$

Calculate the velocity $\boldsymbol{V}_{ocff}$ of the terminal point with Formula (8.2.31), the formula is as follows:

$$\boldsymbol{V}_{ocff} = \boldsymbol{V}_{\text{thrust}} + \boldsymbol{V}_{\text{gravity}} + \boldsymbol{V}_{ocf0} \tag{8.2.60}$$

Because we do not expect the $-K_{\varphi 1}+K_{\varphi 2}t$ and $-K_{\psi 1}+K_{\psi 2}t$ to have any influence on orbital velocity, there is the relationship as follows,

$$\boldsymbol{V}_{ocff} = \boldsymbol{V}_{ocff}\left(\bar{\varphi}_{ocf},\bar{\psi}_{ocf}\right) \tag{8.2.61}$$

That is

$$V_{\text{thrust}}\left(\bar{\varphi}_{ocf}, \bar{\psi}_{ocf}\right) + V_{\text{gravity}}\left(\bar{\varphi}_{ocf}, \bar{\psi}_{ocf}\right) + V_{ocf0} = V_{\text{thrust}} + V_{\text{gravity}} + V_{ocf0}$$

$$(8.2.62)$$

Again,

$$V_{\text{gravity}}\left(\bar{\varphi}_{ocf}, \bar{\psi}_{ocf}\right) = V_{\text{gravity}} \qquad (8.2.63)$$

Hence,

$$V_{\text{thrust}}\left(\bar{\varphi}_{ocf}, \bar{\psi}_{ocf}\right) = V_{\text{thrust}} \qquad (8.2.64)$$

Without considering the constraint of X_{ocff}, here we only consider the second formula and the third formula in scalar form in Formula (8.2.57). The other constrained equations will be given by the position constraint obtained from the second formula in Formula (8.2.64),

$$F0(t_g)K_{\varphi 1} = F1(t_g)K_{\varphi 2} \qquad (8.2.65)$$

From the third formula in Formula (8.2.64), the equation obtained is as follows:

$$F0(t_g)K_{\psi 1} = F1(t_g)K_{\psi 2} \qquad (8.2.66)$$

As a result of Formula (8.2.65), to solve $K_{\varphi 1}$ and $K_{\varphi 2}$, one additional constraint equation is needed. In like manner, to solve $K_{\psi 1}$ and $K_{\psi 2}$, another constraint equation is needed. Following is the process of establishing such two constraint equations.

Firstly, solve the terminal point R_{ocff}, which is integrated twice on Formula (8.2.62), and obtain the formula as follows:

$$R_{ocff} = R_{\text{thrust}} + R_{\text{gravity}} + V_{ocf0} \cdot t_g + R_{ocf0} \qquad (8.2.67)$$

Put Formulas (8.2.39) and (8.2.41) into the above-mentioned formula, and only consider the second formula and the third formula in scalar form in Formula (8.2.67), and obtain the formula as follows:

$$Y_{ocff} = F2(t_g)\sin\left(\bar{\varphi}_{ocf}\right)\cos\left(\bar{\psi}_{ocf}\right) + F2(t_g)K_{\varphi 1}\cos\left(\bar{\varphi}_{ocf}\right)\cos\left(\bar{\psi}_{ocf}\right)$$
$$- F3(t_g)K_{\varphi 2}\cos\left(\bar{\varphi}_{ocf}\right)\cos\left(\bar{\psi}_{ocf}\right) + \frac{1}{2}g_{yocf}t_g^2 + V_{yocf0} \cdot t_g + Y_{ocf0}$$

$$(8.2.68)$$

$$Z_{ocff} = F2(t_g)K_{\psi 1}\cos(\bar{\psi}_{ocf}) - F3(t_g)K_{\psi 2}\cos(\bar{\psi}_{ocf}) + \frac{1}{2}g_{zocf}t_g^2$$
$$+ V_{zocf0} \cdot t_g + Z_{ocf0} \tag{8.2.69}$$

From Formulas (8.2.65) and (8.2.68), we may solve,

$$K_{\varphi 1} = \frac{Y_{ocff} - F2(t_g)\sin(\bar{\varphi}_{ocf})\cos(\bar{\psi}_{ocf}) - \frac{1}{2}g_{yocf}t_g^2 - V_{yocff}\cdot t_g - Y_{ocf0}}{\left(F2(t_g) - \frac{F3(t_g)F0(t_g)}{F1(t_g)}\right)\cos(\bar{\varphi}_{ocf})\cos(\bar{\psi}_{ocf})} \tag{8.2.70}$$

$$K_{\varphi 2} = \frac{\left(Y_{ocff} - F2(t_g)\sin(\bar{\varphi}_{ocf})\cos(\bar{\psi}_{ocf}) - \frac{1}{2}g_{yocf}t_g^2 - V_{yocff}\cdot t_g - Y_{ocf0}\right)\cdot F0(t_g)}{\left(F2(t_g)F1(t_g) - F3(t_g)F0(t_g)\right)\cos(\bar{\varphi}_{ocf})\cos(\bar{\psi}_{ocf})}$$
$$\tag{8.2.71}$$

From Formulas (8.2.66) and (8.2.69), the following equation can be solved as follows:

$$K_{\psi 1} = \frac{Z_{ocff} - \frac{1}{2}g_{zocf}t_g^2 - V_{zocff}\cdot t_g - Z_{ocf0}}{\left(F2(t_g) - \frac{F2(t_g)F0(t_g)}{F1(t_g)}\right)\cos(\bar{\psi}_{ocf})} \tag{8.2.72}$$

$$K_{\psi 2} = \frac{\left(Z_{ocff} - \frac{1}{2}g_{zocf}t_g^2 - V_{zocff}\cdot t_g - Z_{ocf0}\right)\cdot F0(t_g)}{\left(F2(t_g)F1(t_g) - F2(t_g)F0(t_g)\right)\cos(\bar{\psi}_{ocf})} \tag{8.2.73}$$

Formulas (8.2.70)–(8.2.73) are the expression of $K_{\varphi 1}$, $K_{\varphi 2}$, $K_{\psi 1}$, and $K_{\psi 2}$.

To sum up, the blocked diagram of calculating traditional iterative guidance is shown in Fig. 8.7.

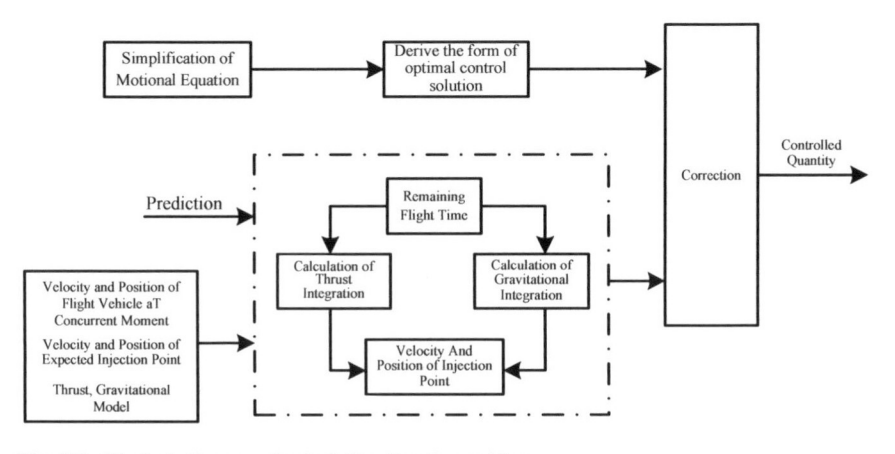

Fig. 8.7 Blocked diagram of calculating iterative guidance

Compared to perturbation guidance, the iterative guidance does not calculate the standard trajectory before launching, which is favorable for shortening the launching time, and is easy for maneuver launching or changing target attacked with larger flexibility. The real-time calculation of trajectory equation on flight vehicle and re-optimization of the flight path have strong adaptability and robustness, with the higher precision of guidance. Main shortcomings of iterative guidance are the complicated equipment, a large quantity of real-time calculation in flight, higher requirements on word length, capacity, and memory capacity of the missile-borne computer. Along with the continuous improvement of capacity and operating speed of the airborne computer, the method of iterative guidance will be increasingly applied in guidance control of modern space technology.

8.2.3   New Direct Guidance Technology

As described in Sect. 8.2.2, the guidance of flight vehicle, in nature, may be regarded as one optimal control problem. Starting from the optimal control principle, choose the appropriate Hamiltonian Functions in accordance with the designated performance parameters and the form of terminal constraint, to derive one group of relations (co-state equation, state equation, control equation, and transversality condition). Then, process such group of equations accordingly, and obtain the command of control angle needed at last. Iterative guidance processes the equation by simplifying the mode of control angle. However, along with the increasingly mature modern numerical solution method and calculating software, the method of direct solutions by transforming the optimal control problem into nonlinear programming problem and obtaining the guidance mode of instructions of control angle is called New Direct Guidance Method.

1. **Convert Optimal Control Problem into Nonlinear Programming Problem**

Commonly, the fundamental ideal of conversion is to divide (share out equally or divide unequally) the whole integration variable (usually the time variable t) to express the continuous state curve and the control quantity curve with the value on the node in the original optimal control problem (that is the discretization, for example, the third-order Simpson Point Collocation, some transformation methods discretize the co-state variables at node). Get the values between nodes through interpolation. Thus, the complicated optimal control problem is transformed into parameter optimization problem.

a. The Third-Order Simpson Point Collocation Method

As for the state equation $\dot{x} = f(t, x, u)$, at any time interval $[t_0, t_f]$, divide such interval into N sections. Each subinterval is

$$[t_i, t_{i+1}], \quad i = 0, 1, 2, \ldots, N - 1 \tag{8.2.74}$$

Let $h_i = t_{i+1} - t_i$, $s = \frac{t - t_i}{h_i}$, $t \in [t_i, t_{i+1}]$, and $s \in [0, 1]$ show any state quantity within such sub-time interval with three times of Hermite Polynomial.

$$x = C_0 + C_1 S + C_2 S^2 + C_3 S^3 \tag{8.2.75}$$

The boundary conditions are,

$$x_1 = x(0), x_2 = x(1), \dot{x}_1 = \left.\frac{dx}{ds}\right|_{s=0}, \dot{x}_2 = \left.\frac{dx}{ds}\right|_{s=1} \tag{8.2.76}$$

To solve and obtain,

$$\begin{bmatrix} C_0 \\ C_1 \\ C_2 \\ C_3 \end{bmatrix} = \begin{bmatrix} 1 & 0 & 0 & 0 \\ 0 & 1 & 0 & 0 \\ -3 & -2 & 3 & -1 \\ 2 & 1 & -2 & 1 \end{bmatrix} \begin{bmatrix} x_1 \\ \dot{x}_1 \\ x_2 \\ \dot{x}_2 \end{bmatrix} \tag{8.2.77}$$

Take the middle of the subinterval $S = 0.5$, put Formula (8.2.77) into Formula (8.2.75) and obtain,

$$x_{c_i} = \frac{x_i + x_{i+1}}{2} + \frac{1}{8} h_i (f_i - f_{i+1})$$
$$\dot{x}_{c_i} = -3 \frac{x_i - x_{i+1}}{2h_i} - \frac{1}{4}(f_i + f_{i+1}) \tag{8.2.78}$$

The third-order Simpson Method takes the state quantity and control quantity of each node as well as the control quantity of collocation point as the variable of optimal decision variable, choose the point collocation as the middle of the subinterval, i.e.,

$$Z = \begin{bmatrix} x_0^T & u_{c_0}^T & u_0^T & \cdots & x_N^T & u_{c_N}^T & u_N^T \end{bmatrix} \tag{8.2.79}$$

Hence, there are $(N+1)(n+m) + m \times N$ decision variables, n is the number of state quantity of each node, and m is the number of control quantity of each node or the point collocation.

The third-order Simpson Method requires the derivative value of point collocation by estimation, i.e., the Formula (8.2.75) should be equal to the derivative value of point collocation obtained by putting Formula (8.2.78) into the state equation. Thus, it could fit the change of optimal state quantity well. Then, there is

$$\varDelta = f_{c_i} + 3\frac{x_i - x_{i+1}}{2h_i} + \frac{1}{4}\left(f_i + f_{i+1}\right) = 0 \qquad (8.2.80)$$

Formula (8.2.80) is called the Hermite–Simpson defect vector. These vectors form the nonlinear equality constraints of the system.

By then, the optimal control problem is transformed into the nonlinear programming problem with constraints. The next work is to search for the optimal value including decision variables with nonlinear programming algorithm, to make the defect vector approach zero, and meet the constraints of control quantity and terminals of the system.

b. Redescribe Trajectory Optimization Problem

With the third-order Simpson point collocation method, transform the optimal control problem into the nonlinear programming problem with equality constraint and inequality constraint.

$$
\begin{aligned}
&\min J(X) \quad X \in R^n \\
&\text{s.t. } g_i(X) \geq 0, \quad i = 1, 2, \ldots, m \\
&\quad\;\; h_j(X) = 0, \quad j = 1, 2, \ldots, l
\end{aligned}
\qquad (8.2.81)
$$

Among which, the $J(X)$ is the performance index, $g_i(X)$ is the inequality constraint, $h_j(X)$ is the equality constraint containing Formula (8.2.78) and terminal constraint.

2. **To Solve Nonlinear Programming Problem**

a. Unconstrained Processing

After processing continuous optimal control model with discretization method, the parameter optimization problem obtained after the transformation is one constrained nonlinear programming problem shown in Formula (8.2.81). Due to the existence of nonlinear constraint, we could not simply use the method of elimination to convert the above-mentioned constraint problems into unconstrained nonlinear problem. The common method is to set up one auxiliary function that takes the descent of the object function and meets the constraint conditions to convert the constraint problem into one unconstrained problem of minimization auxiliary problem. The following describes the issue of solving nonlinear programming problem by applying the Augmented Lagrangian Method.

As for the common minimum problem that contains both inequality constraint and equality constraint, the multiplier penalty function could be defined as follows:

$$L(x, \sigma_k, v_k, \mu_k) = f(x) + \frac{1}{2\sigma_k} \sum_{i=1}^{m} \left\{ \left[\max\left(0, \left(v_i^{(k)} - \sigma_k g_i(x)\right)\right)\right]^2 - \left(v_i^{(k)}\right)^2 \right\}$$

$$+ \frac{\sigma_k}{2} \sum_{i=1}^{l} h_i^2(x) + \sum_{i=1}^{l} \mu_i^{(k)} h_i(x)$$

(8.2.82)

Among which, ω and v are the multiplier vectors of inequality constraint and equality constraint, σ is the penalty factor.

The steps of solving nonlinear programming problem with constraints by the Augmented Lagrangian Method are as follow:

(1) Given the initial point $x^{(0)}$, the equality constrained multiplier vector $v^{(1)}$, inequality constrained multiplier vector $\omega^{(1)}$, penalty factor σ, allowable error ξ, constant $\alpha > 1$, $\beta \in (0, 1)$, and put $k = 1$.
(2) Taking $x^{(k-1)}$ as the initial point, solve the unconstraint optimization problem $\min L(x, \sigma_k, v_k, \mu_k)$ and obtain $x^{(k)}$.
(3) If $\left\| h(x^{(k)}) \right\| < \xi$, then, stop calculating, obtain the optimum solution $x^{(k)}$. Otherwise, go to Step (4).
(4) If $\frac{\left\| h(x^{(k)}) \right\|}{\left\| h(x^{(k-1)}) \right\|} \geq \beta$, put $\sigma = \alpha\sigma$, turn to Step (5); Otherwise, go to Step (5) directly.
(5) Use the following formula to correct the inequality constrained multiplier vector and equality constrained multiplier vector, put $k = k + 1$, and turn to Step (2).

$$\omega_i^{(k+1)} = \max\left(0, \omega_i^{(k)} - \sigma\, g_i\left(x^{(k)}\right)\right)$$
$$v_j^{(k+1)} = v_j^{(k)} - \sigma h_j\left(x^{(k)}\right)$$

(8.2.83)

b. To Solve Unconstrained Optimization Problem

With the Augmented Lagrangian Method, the constrained parameter optimization problem could be transformed into unconstraint one. At present, there are many mature algorithms of solving unconstrained parameter optimization problem. The following is one type of combined variable metric algorithm. The specific steps are as follows:

(1) Given the initial point $x^{(0)}$, the maximum iterative steps N, gradient matrix 2— the norm upper limit ε.
(2) Put $H_1 = I_n$, calculate the gradient matrix $g = \nabla f(x^{(0)})$ at the place of $x^{(0)}$, put $k = 1$.
(3) If meets $\left| \nabla f(x^{(0)}) \right| < \varepsilon$, stop calculating, $x^{(0)}$ is the extreme point; Otherwise, go to Step (4).

(4) Calculate $r = -Hg$, solve $\lambda^* = \arg\min_{\lambda} f(x + \lambda r)$, obtain the optimal step size λ^*. Let $e = x + \lambda^* r$ and calculate $x = x + e$, calculate $g_1 = \nabla f(x)$, $y = g_1 - g$, put $k = k + 1$.

(5) Calculate the gradient $g = \nabla f(x)$. If meets $|\nabla f(x)| < \varepsilon$, stop calculation, obtain the extreme point. If not, turn to Step (6).

(6) If meets $k = N$, then let $x^{(0)} = x^{(k+1)}$, turn to Step (2). If not meet, turn to Step (7).

(7) Calculate $d = Hy$, $a = y^T d$, $b = e^T y$.

(8) If meets $b \geq a$, calculate $H = H + \frac{1}{b}\left[\left(1 + \frac{a}{b}\right)ee^T - ed^T - de^T\right]$. If not meet, calculates $H = H - \frac{1}{a}dd^T + \frac{1}{b}ee^T$. Then, let $g = g_1$, turn to Step (4).

8.3 Transfer Orbit Midcourse Correction Technology

8.3.1 Description of Midcourse Correction

During the process of flight vehicle flying in the transfer orbit, theoretically, as long as relying on the information of initial point and a target point on transfer orbit, calculate and generate the velocity increment needed for transfer, the orbit transfer could be completed. However, due to the affections of nonspherical Earth gravitation, lunisolar attraction, meanwhile, the flight vehicle has the problems of navigation error and deviation of motor thrust, there is an error between the actual transfer orbit and the ideal orbit. Therefore, to ensure the final injection precision of flight vehicle, it is essential to carry out a midcourse correction. The midcourse correction is to correct the orbital deviation aroused by perturbation factors. Try to correct the actual transfer orbit to the nominal transfer orbit, which mainly consists of design stage and execution stage. During the design stage, commonly assume the ideal velocity pulse produced by the midcourse correction motor, further to design the correction point. During the correction stage, commonly use the small motor including attitude control motor to approximately realize the velocity pulse needed.

During the design stage, usually, two correction points shall be calculated, it is shown in Fig. 8.8. Select one appropriate point on the actual and nominal transfer orbit, respectively, which are P_1 and P_2. Then, design one orbit that crosses through the two points, which is used as one middle transitional orbit that connects the actual and nominal transfer orbit. The flight vehicle applies pulse when it starts sliding freely to Point P_1 from the actual transfer orbit. After that, it enters into the transitional orbit and keeps on sliding freely. When slides to point P_2, it applies velocity pulse again and enters into the nominal orbit. From this we can see, two corrections have been applied during the process from the actual transfer orbit to nominal transfer orbit.

The two midcourse correction methods, first of all, shall determine the Point P_1 on actual transfer orbit and Point P_2 on nominal transfer orbit. Once such two points

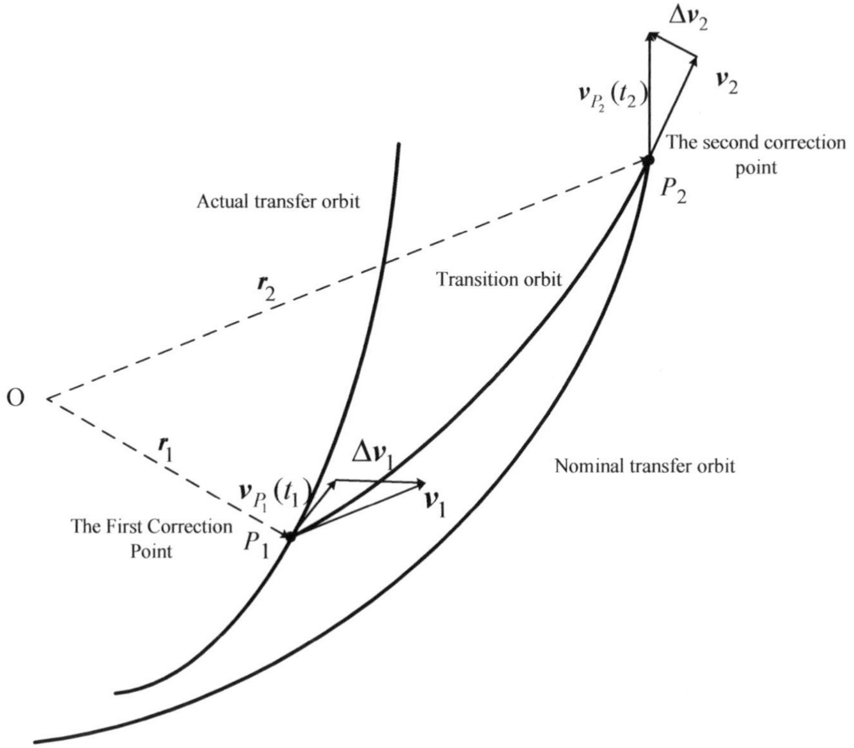

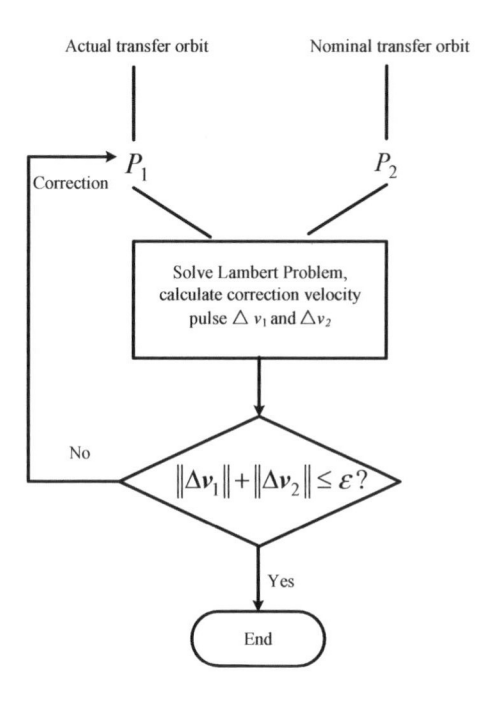

Fig. 8.8 Schematic diagram of two midcourse corrections

Fig. 8.9 Schematic diagram of determining Point P_1 and P_2

are decided, the remaining key point lays on designing one transitional orbit that crosses through Point P_1 and Point P_2. After the transition track is determined, its velocities at Point P_1 and Point P_2 are determined. Assume it is v_1 and v_2, the velocity of the actual transfer orbit at Point P_1 is $v_{P_1}(t_1)$, the velocity of nominal transfer orbit at Point P_2 is $v_{P_2}(t_2)$.

Under the assumption of ideal velocity pulse model, the velocity pulse of flight vehicle applied at Point P_1 $\Delta v_1 = v_1 - v_{P_1}(t_1)$, it enters into transition track from the actual transfer track. After that, the flight vehicle applies velocity pulse $\Delta v_2 = v_{P_2}(t_2) - v_2$ when slides to Point P_2.

The determination of correction points P_1 and P_2 needs one iterative calculation process. Specifically, given the initial values of Point P_1 and P_2, calculate the velocity pulse needed for correction by solving Lambert Problem (given the position vector and transfer time of two points in space related to the attraction center, determine the transition track that crosses the two points). Then, return to correct the P_1 and P_2 according to the amplitudes of velocity pulse until they meet the requirements, it is shown in Fig. 8.9. Here, ε is the upper limit of the amplitude of the scheduled velocity pulse.

8.3.2   Strategy of Midcourse Correction

This Section mainly discusses the two midcourse correction plans on the basis of solving Lambert Problem. The specific solution of Lambert Problem refers to the related information.

Known from Fig. 8.8, the selection of initial point and the target point of midcourse correction are not fixed. The starting point shall be on the actual transfer orbit, and the target point shall be on the nominal transfer orbit, the target point shall have sufficient distance from the next orbital maneuver. Therefore, the next consideration is how to select the initial point and target point, to minimize the cost of midcourse correction, i.e., the amplitude of velocity pulse shall be minimized.

Since the data of position and velocity of the actual and nominal transfer orbit are known, if the passage time t_1 and t_2 are given, the position vector of the initial and terminal ends could be determined by numerical integration or the perturbation of orbital elements, that is the position vectors of initial point and target point. Hence, it follows that the time at the beginning of the end is the variable-free parameter. As for midcourse correction, save energy as possible under the premise of meeting the accuracy of correction, i.e., the volume of velocity pulse. Hence, commonly, the velocity pulses needed for correction is taken as the performance index. After the partial derivative expressions of the performance index of applying velocity pulse corresponding to the endpoint are given, respectively, with the state transfer matrix and classical variational principle.

Assume $X(t)$ is the state trajectory corresponding to certain track, and defines $M = X(t_0)$ and $N = X(t_1)$. Thus, the values of M, N are related to the selection of

Fig. 8.10 Schematic diagram of asynchronous variation

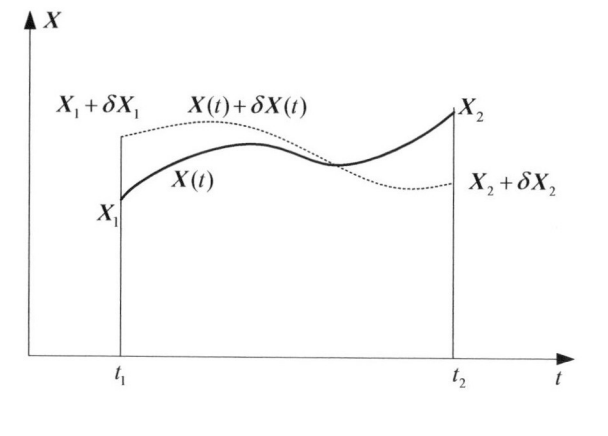

Fig. 8.11 Schematic diagram of moving boundary variation

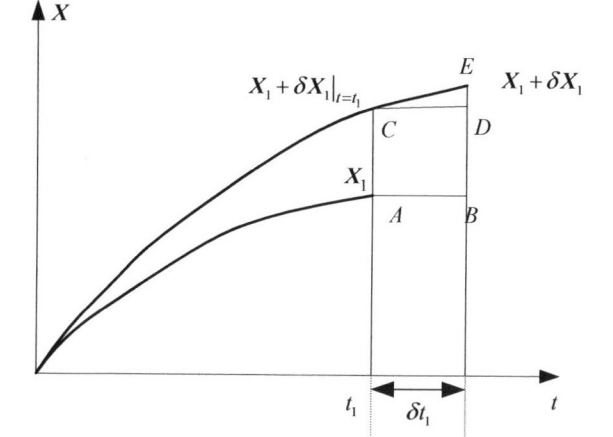

state trajectory $X(t)$ that is M, N are the function of $X(t)$, while $X(t)$ is the argument of M, N. Assume the state track has tiny change that is $X(t) + \delta X(t)$ then the function M, N will change either. δX_0, δX_1 are defined as the variations of M, N, then, the state trajectory as shown in Fig. 8.10.

The state transfer matrix may describe the variation relations of M, N. The state transfer matrix in the Two-Body Problem has the analytical expressions. The state transfer matrix of track in N-body Problem may be solved through numerical method. From the nature of state matrix, obtain,

$$\begin{cases} \delta r_2 = \boldsymbol{\Phi}_{rr}\delta r_1 + \boldsymbol{\Phi}_{rv}\delta v_1 \\ \delta v_2 = \boldsymbol{\Phi}_{vr}\delta r_1 + \boldsymbol{\Phi}_{vv}\delta v_1 \end{cases} \tag{8.3.1}$$

Here, the $\boldsymbol{\Phi}_{rr}, \boldsymbol{\Phi}_{rv}, \boldsymbol{\Phi}_{vr}, \boldsymbol{\Phi}_{vv}$ corresponds to the four parts of $\delta r, \delta v$.

Formula (8.3.1) describes the influence of tiny change of initial state on the state of termination. With Formula (8.3.1), solve the δv_1 and δv_2, the specific forms are as follow:

$$\begin{cases} \delta v_1 = F\delta r_1 + E\delta r_2 \\ \delta v_2 = H\delta r_1 + G\delta r_2 \end{cases} \tag{8.3.2}$$

Here, $E = \boldsymbol{\Phi}_{\mathrm{rv}}^{-1}, F = -\boldsymbol{\Phi}_{\mathrm{rv}}^{-1}\boldsymbol{\Phi}_{\mathrm{rr}}, G = \boldsymbol{\Phi}_{\mathrm{vv}}\boldsymbol{\Phi}_{\mathrm{rv}}^{-1}, H = \boldsymbol{\Phi}_{\mathrm{vr}} - \boldsymbol{\Phi}_{\mathrm{vv}}\boldsymbol{\Phi}_{\mathrm{rv}}^{-1}\boldsymbol{\Phi}_{\mathrm{rr}}$.

The above-mentioned conclusions are derived on the basis of asynchronous variation, i.e., to meet $\delta t = 0$ for all the time. Because the moments of applying pulses for two times during the process of optimization are the free adjustable parameters, the analysis of the conditions of moving boundary variation follows. To show the difference between equal time edge and moving boundary variation clearly, Formula (8.3.2) is rewritten as follows:

$$\begin{cases} \delta v_1|_{t=t_1} = F\delta r_1|_{t=t_1} + E\delta r_1|_{t=t_2} \\ \delta v_2|_{t=t_2} = H\delta r_1|_{t=t_1} + G\delta r_1|_{t=t_2} \end{cases} \tag{8.3.3}$$

Next, analyze the moving boundary variation. If the time endpoint t_1 is no longer fixed, but have one tiny change δt_1, the change of state track is shown in Fig. 8.11.

The Segment AC in Fig. 8.11 corresponds to asynchronous variation $\delta X_1|_{t=t_1}$, while Segment BE corresponds to moving boundary variation δX_1. If the change of boundary δt_1 is very less, approximate relations may be derived as follows:

$$\delta X_1 \approx \delta X_1|_{t=t_1} + \frac{dX}{dt}\bigg|_{t=t_1}\delta t_1 \tag{8.3.4}$$

Derive the relations between the moving boundary variation of flight vehicle state variables r, v and the moments t_0, t_1 of asynchronous variation at the two endpoints with Formula (8.3.11),

$$\begin{cases} \delta r_1 = \delta r_1|_{t=t_1} + v_1\delta t_1 \\ \delta r_2 = \delta r_2|_{t=t_2} + v_2\delta t_2 \end{cases} \tag{8.3.5}$$

Here, v_1, v_2 are related to the velocity of flight vehicle at the moments t_1, t_2, the variation of velocity may be shown as follows:

$$\begin{cases} \delta v_1 = \delta v_1|_{t=t_1} + a_1\delta t_1 \\ \delta v_2 = \delta v_2|_{t=t_2} + a_2\delta t_2 \end{cases} \tag{8.3.6}$$

Here, a_1, a_2 are the acceleration of flight vehicle related to the moments of t_0, t_1

From Formulas (8.3.3), (8.3.5), and (8.3.6) solve the expressions of velocity variations at two endpoints under the conditions of boundary disturbance,

Fig. 8.12 The state trajectory
whose two ends constrained
by ephemeris

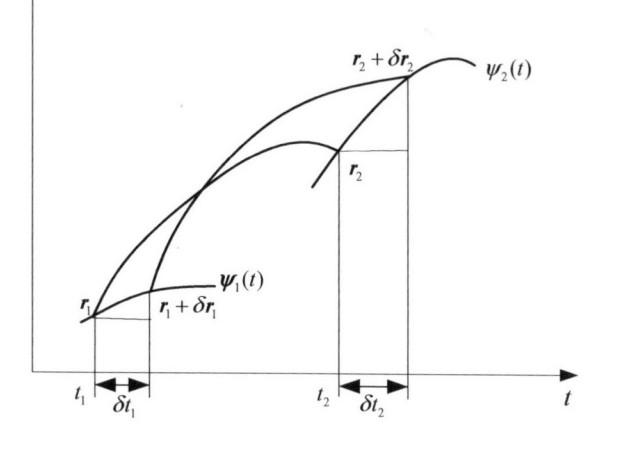

$$\begin{cases} \delta v_1|_{t=t_1} = F(\delta r_1 - v_1 \delta t_1) + a_1 \delta t_1 + E(\delta r_2 - v_2 \delta t_2) \\ \delta v_2|_{t=t_2} = H(\delta r_1 - v_1 \delta t_1) + a_2 \delta t_2 + G(\delta r_2 - v_2 \delta t_2) \end{cases} \tag{8.3.7}$$

In analyzing the midcourse correction of transfer orbit, the points on actual transfer orbit and nominal transfer orbit could be taken as the mass points in space that move in respective ephemeris. Thus, r_1, r_2 shall meet the following relations,

$$\begin{cases} r_1(t) = \psi_1(t) \\ r_2(t) = \psi_2(t) \end{cases} \tag{8.3.8}$$

Here, ψ_1 is the ephemeris of actual transfer orbit, and ψ_2 is the ephemeris of nominal transfer orbit. The state trajectory of the two endpoints constrained by ephemeris is shown in Fig. 8.12.

From Fig. 8.12 one can see, the r_1 and r_2 shall correspond to and meet the following expressions,

$$\begin{cases} \delta r_1 \approx \dfrac{d\psi_1(t)}{dt}\bigg|_{t=t_1} \delta t_1 \\ \delta r_2 \approx \dfrac{d\psi_2(t)}{dt}\bigg|_{t=t_2} \delta t_2 \end{cases} \tag{8.3.9}$$

The $\dfrac{d\psi_1(t)}{dt}\bigg|_{t=t_1}$ and $\dfrac{d\psi_2(t)}{dt}\bigg|_{t=t_2}$ in Eq. (8.3.9) are the respective velocity $v_{P_1}(t_1)$ of the actual orbit at the moment of t_1 and the velocity $v_{P_2}(t_2)$ of nominal orbit at the moment of t_2, Eq. (8.3.9) may be recorded as

$$\begin{cases} \delta \boldsymbol{r}_1 \approx \boldsymbol{v}_{P_1}(t_1)\delta t_1 \\ \delta \boldsymbol{r}_2 \approx \boldsymbol{v}_{P_2}(t_2)\delta t_2 \end{cases} \tag{8.3.10}$$

Put Eq. (8.3.10) into Eq. (8.3.2) to obtain the following,

$$\begin{cases} \delta \boldsymbol{v}_1 = [\boldsymbol{F}(\boldsymbol{v}_{P_1}(t_1) - \boldsymbol{v}_1) + \boldsymbol{a}_1]\delta t_1 + \boldsymbol{E}(\boldsymbol{v}_{P_2}(t_2) - \boldsymbol{v}_2)\delta t_2 \\ \delta \boldsymbol{v}_2 = \boldsymbol{H}(\boldsymbol{v}_{P_1}(t_1) - \boldsymbol{v}_1)\delta t_1 + [\boldsymbol{a}_2 + \boldsymbol{G}(\boldsymbol{v}_{P_2}(t_2) - \boldsymbol{v}_2)]\delta t_2 \end{cases} \tag{8.3.11}$$

From Eq. (8.3.11), derive the partial derivative corresponding to the following velocity:

$$\begin{cases} \frac{\partial \boldsymbol{v}_1}{\partial t_1} = \boldsymbol{F}(\boldsymbol{v}_{P_1}(t_1) - \boldsymbol{v}_1) + \boldsymbol{a}_1 \\ \frac{\partial \boldsymbol{v}_1}{\partial t_2} = \boldsymbol{E}(\boldsymbol{v}_{P_2}(t_2) - \boldsymbol{v}_2) \\ \frac{\partial \boldsymbol{v}_2}{\partial t_1} = \boldsymbol{H}(\boldsymbol{v}_{P_1}(t_1) - \boldsymbol{v}_1) \\ \frac{\partial \boldsymbol{v}_2}{\partial t_2} = \boldsymbol{a}_2 + \boldsymbol{G}(\boldsymbol{v}_{P_2}(t_2) - \boldsymbol{v}_2) \end{cases} \tag{8.3.12}$$

Commonly, the performance index of two-pulse correction flying from the actual orbit to nominal orbit could be shown as follows:

$$J = \sqrt{\|\boldsymbol{v}_1 - \boldsymbol{v}_{P_1}(t_1)\|^2} + \sqrt{\|\boldsymbol{v}_2 - \boldsymbol{v}_{P_2}(t_2)\|^2} \tag{8.3.13}$$

For the convenience of investigating the partial derivative of performance index related to the moments of t_1 and t_2, select the performance index as

$$J_1 = J^2 = [\boldsymbol{v}_1 - \boldsymbol{v}_{P_1}(t_1)]^{\mathrm{T}}[\boldsymbol{v}_1 - \boldsymbol{v}_{P_1}(t_1)] + [\boldsymbol{v}_2 - \boldsymbol{v}_{P_2}(t_2)]^{\mathrm{T}}[\boldsymbol{v}_2 - \boldsymbol{v}_{P_2}(t_2)] \tag{8.3.14}$$

Thus, the partial derivative of the total velocity increment related to the starting moment of correction is

$$\frac{\partial J_1}{\partial t_1} = \frac{\partial J_1}{\partial \boldsymbol{v}_1} \frac{\partial \boldsymbol{v}_1}{\partial t_1} + \frac{\partial J_1}{\partial \boldsymbol{v}_{P_1}(t_1)} \frac{\partial \boldsymbol{v}_{P_1}(t_1)}{\partial t_1} + \frac{\partial J_1}{\partial \boldsymbol{v}_2} \frac{\partial \boldsymbol{v}_2}{\partial t_1} + \frac{\partial J_1}{\partial \boldsymbol{v}_{P_2}(t_2)} \frac{\partial \boldsymbol{v}_{P_2}(t_2)}{\partial t_1} \tag{8.3.15}$$

Put the partial derivatives in Eq. (8.3.12) into Eq. (8.3.15) to obtain,

$$\frac{\partial J_1}{\partial t_1} = 2[\boldsymbol{v}_1 - \boldsymbol{v}_{P_1}(t_1)]^{\mathrm{T}}\boldsymbol{F}(\boldsymbol{v}_{P_1}(t_1) - \boldsymbol{v}_1) + 2[\boldsymbol{v}_2 - \boldsymbol{v}_{P_2}(t_2)]^{\mathrm{T}}\boldsymbol{H}(\boldsymbol{v}_{P_1}(t_1) - \boldsymbol{v}_1) \tag{8.3.16}$$

$$\frac{\partial J_1}{\partial t_2} = 2[\boldsymbol{v}_1 - \boldsymbol{v}_{P_1}(t_1)]^{\mathrm{T}}\boldsymbol{E}(\boldsymbol{v}_{P_2}(t_2) - \boldsymbol{v}_2) + 2[\boldsymbol{v}_2 - \boldsymbol{v}_{P_2}(t_2)]^{\mathrm{T}}\boldsymbol{G}(\boldsymbol{v}_{P_2}(t_2) - \boldsymbol{v}_2) \tag{8.3.17}$$

With such two derivatives and Newton Iteration Method, the midcourse correction of the two-pulse transfer orbits with free time of the endpoints, the steps of solution are as follows:

(1) Given the initial departure and arrival moment t_1, t_2, calculate the positions r_1, r_2, and the flight speed $v_{P_1}(t_1)$, $v_{P_2}(t_2)$ of the actual orbit and nominal orbit.
(2) Solve the related Lambert problems, and obtain the speed v_1, v_2 related to the flight vehicle at the initial and terminal moments.
(3) Solve the state transfer matrix of such orbit section, and obtain E, F, G, and H.
(4) From Eqs. (8.3.16) and (8.3.17), solve the partial derivative of the target function to the initial moment and terminal moment.
(5) Use Newton Iterative to correct the initial moment and terminal moment, and repeat (1)–(5) until it reaches to the precision required.

In Step (5), use Newton Iterative Method to correct the initial moment t_1 and terminal moment t_2, substantially, it is equal to solving the equation set $\frac{\partial J_1}{\partial t_1} = \frac{\partial J_1}{\partial t_2} = 0$, let $f_1 = \frac{\partial J_1}{\partial t_1}$, $f_2 = \frac{\partial J_1}{\partial t_2}$, the iterative calculation needs to obtain four derivatives $\frac{\partial f_1}{\partial t_1}$, $\frac{\partial f_1}{\partial t_2}$, $\frac{\partial f_2}{\partial t_1}$, and $\frac{\partial f_2}{\partial t_2}$. Although the analytical expressions of f_1 and f_2 are obtained from Eqs. (8.3.16) and (8.3.17), the nature of partial derivative of state transfer matrix to be analyzed in solving the calculation process of partial derivatives could be known in analyzing the forms of the expressions, specifically, the derivation will be more complicated. Therefore, in actual calculation, the difference quotient algorithm could be used for approximately calculating the values of the four partial derivatives $\frac{\partial f_1}{\partial t_1}$, $\frac{\partial f_1}{\partial t_2}$, $\frac{\partial f_2}{\partial t_1}$, and $\frac{\partial f_2}{\partial t_2}$. This will not affect the speed and effects of iterative calculation. For example, $\frac{\partial f_1}{\partial t_1} \approx \frac{f_1(t_1 + \Delta t_1, t_2) - f_1(t_1, t_2)}{\Delta t_1}$, Δt_1 may take a small enough positive number. In addition, set up the upper limit of iterative times for the solving process, to avoid the over more iterative calculation steps.

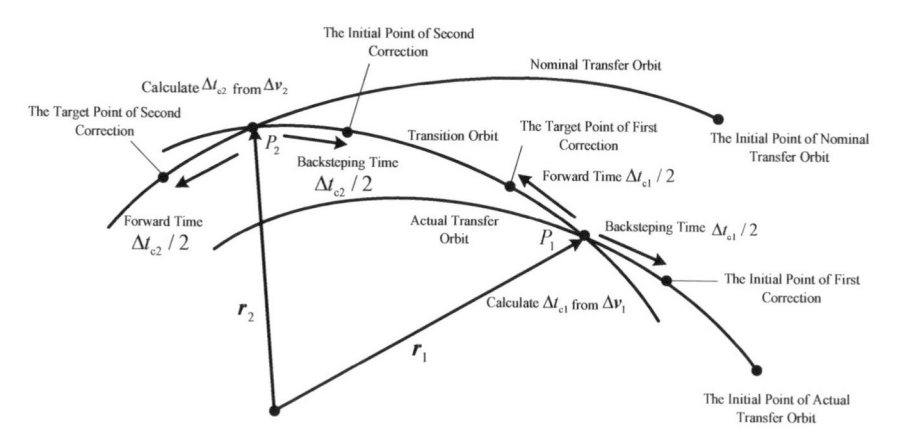

Fig. 8.13 Calculate the two corrections, i.e., initial point and target point

8.3.3 Illustration on Actual Execution of Midcourse Correction

The previous Sects. 8.3.1 and 8.3.2 have discussed the plan of obtaining two correction speed pulses on the basis of solving Lambert problem and minimize the amplitude of pulse correction by moving boundary variation and further adjustment of flight time. Finally, obtain the optimized correction speed pulse.

After obtaining the two corrected speed pulses Δv_1 and Δv_2, the next step is to approximately realize the needed speed pulse with a small motor. It is shown in Fig. 8.13.

First of all, in accordance with the following formula,

$$\Delta t = \frac{m_0 I_{sp}}{F}\left[1 - \exp(-\frac{\|\Delta v\|}{I_{sp}})\right] \tag{8.3.18}$$

Calculate the two engine start time Δt_{c1} and Δt_{c2} with Δv_1 and Δv_2. Among which, the thrust F and specific thrust I_{sp} are the respective thrust and specific thrust of the small motor. Taking the position and speed of actual transfer orbit at the moment of $t_1 - \Delta t_{c1}/2$ as the one-time correction startup point (initial point), and taking the position and speed of the transfer orbit at the moment of $t_2 - \Delta t_{c2}/2$ as the second correction startup point (target point). The thrust direction is always along Δv_1. Take the position and speed of transition orbit at the moment of $t_2 - \Delta t_{c2}/2$ as the second correction startup point (initial point), and the position and speed of nominal orbit at the moment of $t_2 + \Delta t_{c2}/2$ as the second correction shutdown point (object point) the thrust direction is always along the Δv_2. When the flight vehicle arrives at the correction starting point, the small motor starts ignition and correcting, the durations of ignition are, respectively, Δt_{c1} and Δt_{c2}.

8.4 Analysis of Simulation Results

The data of launching point and data of Earth reference ellipsoidal model are the same as that in Chap. 5. The initial mass of flight vehicle in guidance and midcourse correction simulation are 8680.5548 kg, the thrust of sustainer motor is 6500 N, the specific thrust is 3095.00 k/s, the thrust of the small motor is 600 N, and the specific thrust is 2150.00 m/s.

8.4.1 Simulation of Iterative Guidance

In launching inertial system, the initial position vector of flight vehicle is $[-550938.9793, -13025658.6429, -261167.0713]^T$ m, the velocity vector is

Fig. 8.14 Schematic diagram
of remaining time

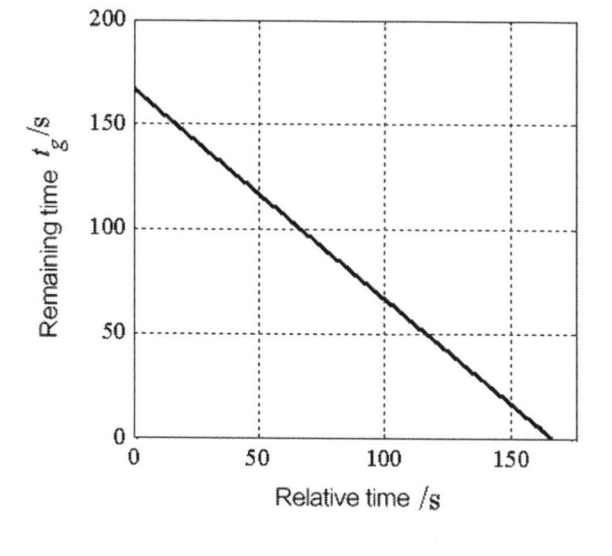

Fig. 8.15 Schematic diagram
of pitch angle command φ

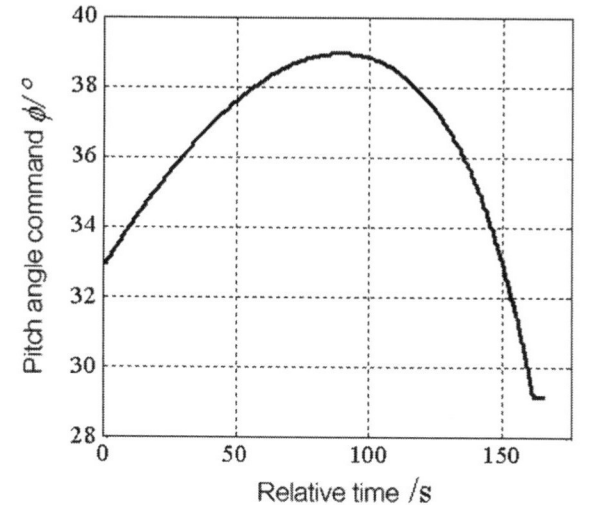

$[-7707.1634, 626.3898, 55.7839]^{\mathrm{T}}$ m/s, the position vector of objective point in
geocentric inertial system is $[3508767.9154, -5592988.0826, -935519.0450]^{\mathrm{T}}$ m,
velocity vector is $[5275.7779, 2620.4544, 4890.2614]^{\mathrm{T}}$ m/s, transfer the position
and velocity of objective point into the orbital coordinate system of injection point,
the corresponding position vector is $[0, 6668445.3855, 0]^{\mathrm{T}}$ m, velocity vector is
$[7655.3005, -107.9146, 0]^{\mathrm{T}}$ m/s, simulate the iterative guidance method introduced
in Sect. 9.2.2 to fulfill the thrust needed for guidance by sustainer motor. The
change of attitude angle is realized by the attitude control motor. During the process
of guidance, the geocentric angle is taken as fixed value, when the remaining time is

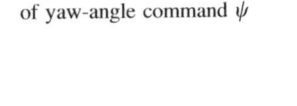

Fig. 8.16 Schematic diagram of yaw-angle command ψ

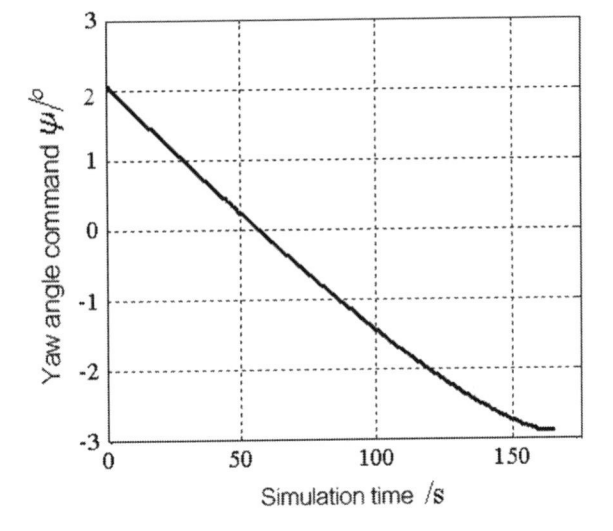

Fig. 8.17 Schematic of position deviation in X-direction

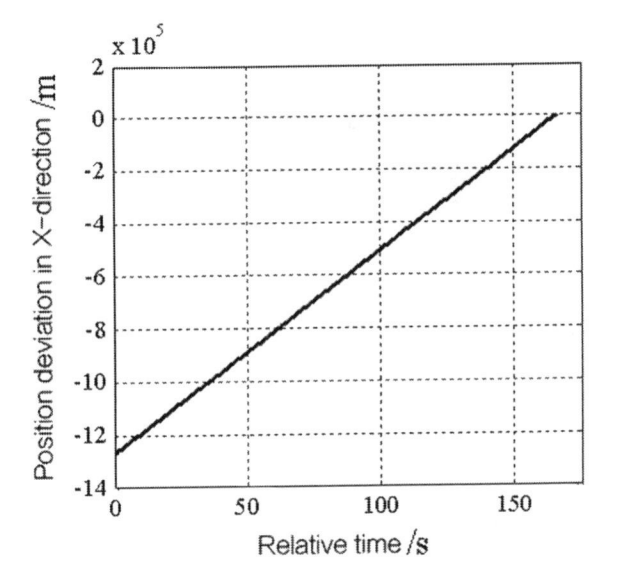

less than 5 s, stop the iterative calculation (that is the command of attitude angle takes constant) of command of attitude angle. The simulation results refer to Figs. 8.14, 8.15, 8.16, 8.17, 8.18, 8.19, 8.20, 8.21, and 8.22. Among which, the command of pitch angle and yaw angle are described related to launching inertial system, the position and velocity deviation are described in relation to orbital coordinate system of the injection point.

Known from the above-mentioned simulation results, during the whole process of guidance, the remaining time is gradually reduced to zero, the error of position

Fig. 8.18 Schematic diagram
of position in *Y*-direction

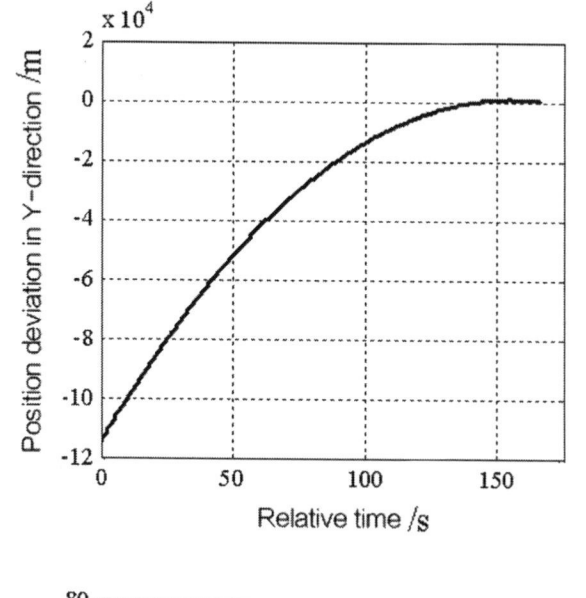

Fig. 8.19 Schematic of
position deviation in
Z-direction

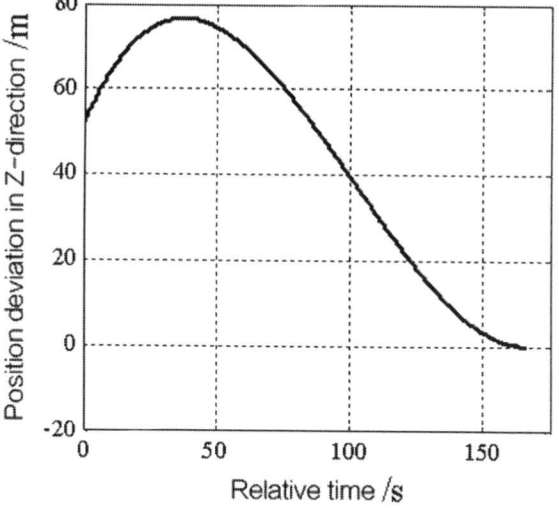

Fig. 8.20 Schematic diagram
of speed deviation
in *X*-direction

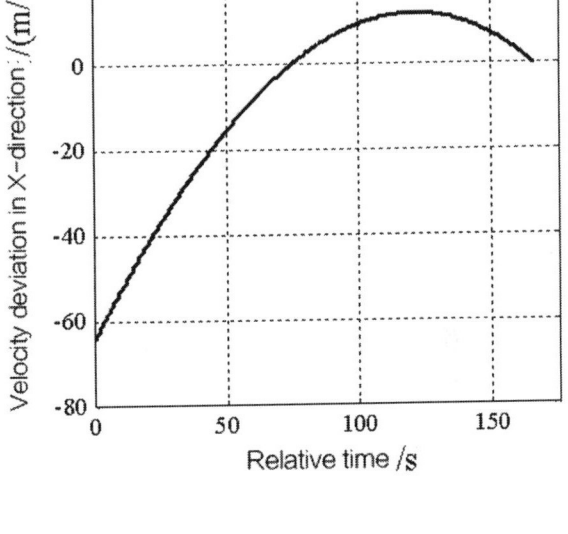

Fig. 8.21 Schematic diagram
of speed deviation
in *Y*-direction

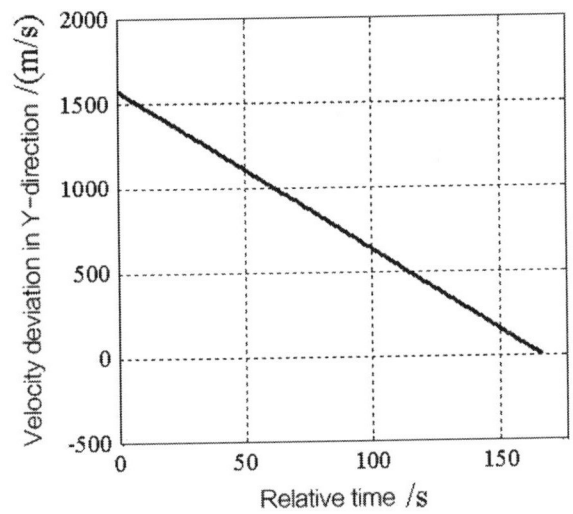

and velocity in three directions approach to zero finally. After the guidance ends,
the position and velocity deviation in the orbital coordinate system of injection
point refer to Table 8.1.

The combined results in Tables 8.1, 8.2, and 8.3, and Table 8.1 shows the
effectiveness of iterative guidance method, which could meet the requirement of
precision of final injection.

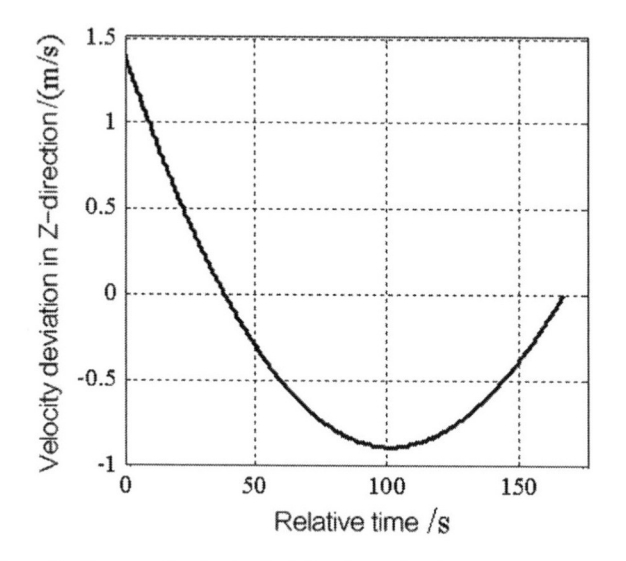

Fig. 8.22 Schematic diagram of velocity deviation in Z-direction

Table 8.1 Deviation of guidance position and velocity

Deviation of position from target point (m)			Deviation of velocity from target point (m/s)		
X	Y	Z	V_x	V_y	V_z
35.7889	−0.0325	−0.0061	0.0498	−0.0465	−0.0036

Table 8.2 Parameters of two midcourse corrections

	The first correction point	The second correction point
Velocity difference at *Intersection Point* (m/s)	3.0234	2.5915
Ignition time of attitud control motor (s)	43.7113	37.4169

Table 8.3 Deviation after two midcourse corrections

Deviation data	Deviation of position from target point correction point (m)			Deviation of velocity from target correction point (m/s)		
	X	Y	Z	V_x	V_y	V_z
The 1st	−22.4457	10.7946	−7.8382	0.0259	−0.0014	0.0153
The 2nd	38.9995	40.3440	47.8097	−0.0511	0.0673	0.0065

8.4.2 Simulation of Midcourse Correction

In launching inertial system, assume the initial position of actual transfer orbit is $[1865014.8, 40816.2, 150433.5]^T$ m, velocity is $[7412.601, -2160.522, -130.991]^T$ m/s, the position of initial point of nominal transfer orbit is $[2405429.8, -141936.2, 140275.6]^T$ m, velocity is $[7201.003, -2784.509, -146.536]^T$ m/s, simulate the strategy of midcourse correction discussed in Sect. 8.3, provide the thrust needed for guidance by small motor, first, calculate the parameters of two midcourse corrections, and obtain the following table.

From Table 8.2 we could know that the ignition time of small motor is within the allowable range. The position and velocity deviation corrected (described in geocentric inertial system) refer to Table 8.3.

Known from the data in Table 8.3, after the second midcourse correction, the position deviation from the target point is 73.7182 m and the velocity deviation is 0.0848 m/s. After two midcourse corrections, the actual transfer orbit could be corrected to near the nominal orbit, which provides good initial conditions for the following transfer mission.

Reference Documentation

1. Song, Zhengyu. 2014. *Design of Control System of High Reliability Launch Vehicle*. China Astronautic Publishing House.
2. Zhang, Libing. 2010. *Rocket Upper Stage Navigation, Research on Midcourse Correction and Attitude Control*. Harbin Institute of Technology.
3. Zeng, Guoqiang. 2000. *Research on Dynamic of Orbits and Guidance Methods of Lunar Probe*. National University of Defense Technology.
4. Yuan, Jianping, Yushan Zhao. 2014. *Design of Flight Vehicle Deep Space Flight Trajectory*. China Astronautic Publishing House.
5. Cui, Pingyuan, Dong Qiao, Gutao Cui. 2013. *Design and Optimization of Deep Space Exploration Orbit*. Science Press.
6. Lu, P., S. Forbes, and M. Baldwin. 2012. A Versatile Powered Guidance Algorithm. In *AIAA Guidance, Navigation, and Control Conference*, 4843.
7. Yang, Jiachi, Qinhong Fang, Yuntong Zhong, Weilian Yang, Shuqing Chen. 1999. *Dynamics of Orbits and Control of Aircraft: (First Volume)*. China Astronautic Publishing House.
8. Yang, Jiachi, Qinghong Fan, Yuntong Zhang. 2001. *Dynamics of Orbits and Control of Aircraft: (Second Volume)*. China Astronautic Publishing House.
9. Zhang, Renwei. 1998. *Dynamics of Attitude and Control of Satellite Orbit*. Beihang University Press.
10. Wang, Mengyi, Yong Jiang. 2008. Research on Midcourse Correction of Transfer Track for Near-Ground Vehicle . In *2008 Proceedings of The National Doctoral Forum 2008 (Aeronautical and Astronautical Science and Technology*, 312–323.
11. Chen, Shinian. *Design of Control System*.

Chapter 9
Orbital Control Strategy

9.1 Introduction

The previous chapters have discussed the orbital prediction technology, inertial navigation and initial alignment technologies, inertial/satellite integrated navigation technology, inertial/starlight integrated navigation technology, inertial device redundant fault tolerance and fault reconfiguration technology, and guidance and midcourse correction technology of the OTV. During the whole process of flight mission of OTV, the technologies described in these chapters will be involved. Thus, the chapter takes the example of OTV sending the payloads into Earth synchronous orbit to make one integrated description of the technical applications in the chapters.

The whole flight process is shown in Figs. 9.1 and 9.2.

From Figs. 9.1 and 9.2, we could know that after the vehicle completes the preparation works such as initial alignment, the base rocket that hosts the OTV and the payload is launched from Point A on the Earth. The rocket puts the flight vehicle and payloads into parking orbit after one flight starting from takeoff. The rocket separates from the flight vehicle and payloads at the Point B of the parking orbit. From then on, the vehicle will slide freely with the payloads on the parking orbit; this is the first free sliding of the whole flight process. When vehicle slides to Point C of the parking orbit, it carries out the first ignition guidance.

After the guidance ends, theoretically, from the Point D, the flight vehicle will enter one nominal transfer orbit designed in advance. However, due to the existence of nonspherical Earth gravity and guidance deviation, the actual transfer orbit entered by the flight vehicle and the nominal transfer orbit deviate, and along with the increasing of time, the deviation will be increasingly large, which leads to the failure of scheduled maneuver mission; the payloads could not be put into the geostationary orbit finally. Therefore, during the section of transfer orbit, midcourse correction is needed. Carrying out the midcourse correction twice with the nominal orbital control method, the Point E on transfer orbit is taken as the starting point of

© Springer Nature Singapore Pte Ltd. and National Defense Industry Press, Beijing 2018
X. Li and C. Li, *Navigation and Guidance of Orbital Transfer Vehicle*, Navigation:
Science and Technology, https://doi.org/10.1007/978-981-10-6334-3_9

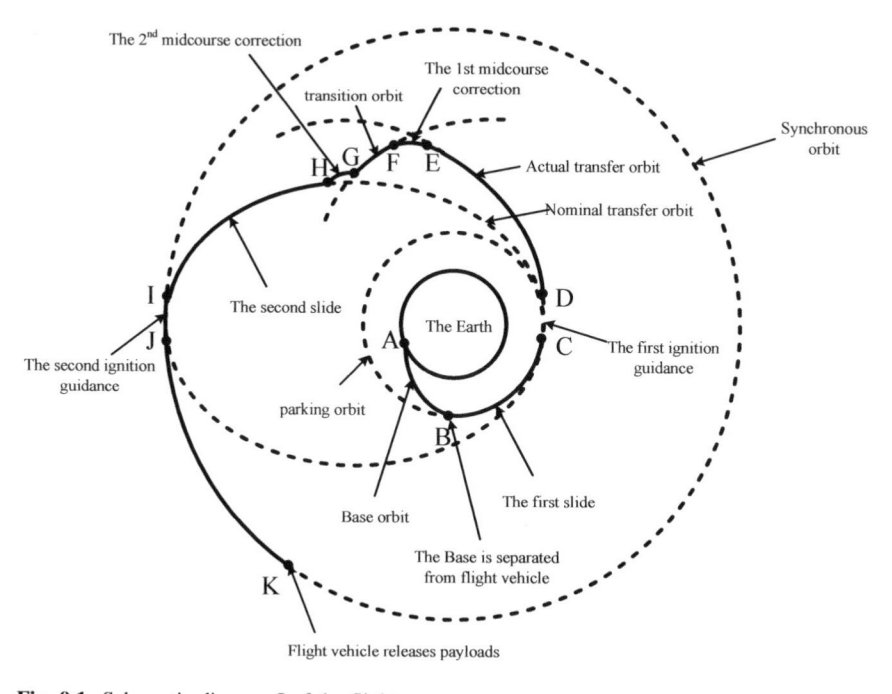

Fig. 9.1 Schematic diagram I of the flight process

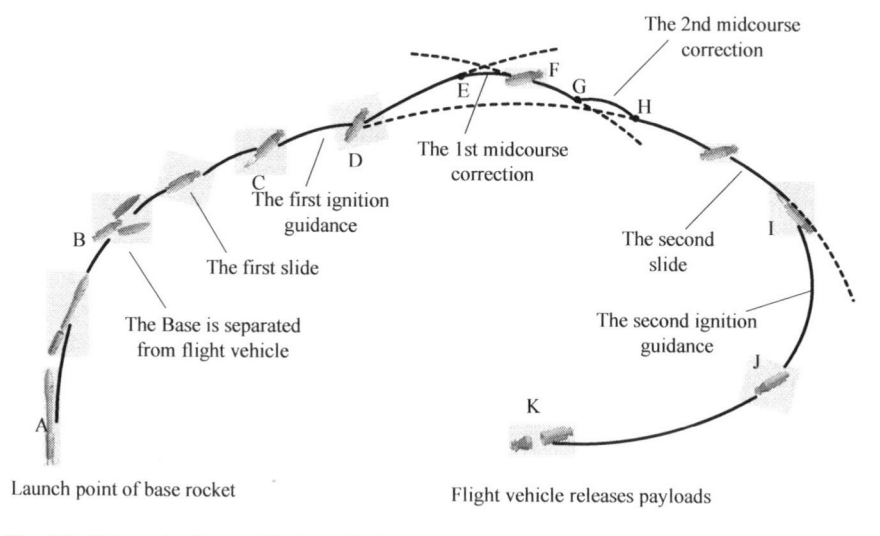

Fig. 9.2 Schematic diagram II of the flight process

midcourse correction. After the first midcourse correction, it enters the Point F of the transfer orbit. After that, the flight vehicle slides to Point G of the transition orbit and carries out the second midcourse correction. After the correction is completed, the flight vehicle enters into the Point H of the nominal transfer orbit and starts the second free sliding of the whole flight process (without considering the slide during the process of midcourse correction). When the flight vehicle slides to Point I of the nominal transfer orbit, it carries out the second ignition guidance. After the guidance is completed, it enters into Point J of the geostationary orbit. Ever since the flight vehicle will release the payloads when slides to Point K on the synchronous orbit, the whole flight mission is completed.

The whole flight process may be divided into the following sections:

1. The base rocket hosting the flight vehicle and payloads flies to Point B of the parking orbit from Point A on ground, and separates from the flight vehicle and payloads at Point B.
2. The flight vehicle enters parking orbit from Point B by hosting the payloads. After the first free sliding, it carries out the first ignition guidance at Point C of the parking orbit. After the guidance is completed, due to the error, the flight vehicle enters actual transfer orbit.
3. The flight vehicle carries out the first midcourse correction at Point E of the actual transfer orbit. After that, it enters Point F of transition orbit.
4. The flight vehicle carries out the second midcourse correction when slides to Point G of transition orbit. After that, it enters Point H of the nominal transfer orbit.
5. The flight vehicle starts the second free slide. When it slides to Point I of nominal transfer orbit, it carries out the second ignition brake. After the guidance ends, it enters Point I of the synchronous orbit.
6. The flight vehicle slides to Point K on the synchronous orbit and releases the payloads.

In this chapter, we will discuss the above-mentioned flight process as an example to describe the specific application of the contents described in the previous chapters.

9.2 Orbital Control Strategy

9.2.1 Design of Initial Alignment

Before starting the flight missions, the OTV is hosted in the base rocket with the payloads. Because the navigation system of the OTV is independent of the base rocket, there is no information exchange. Before the base rocket takes off from Point A on ground, the INS of the OTV shall fulfill the initial alignment. Considering the autonomy and universality of the flight vehicle, the autonomous alignment mode is used. The main factors to be taken into consideration during design process are as follows.

1. Selection of alignment method

In views of the advantages of alignment accuracy and rapidity based on the inertial system, digital filter could reduce the effects of jamming signals and the alignment technology based on inertial system could be used for initial alignment for the INS of the OTV.

2. Digital Filter Processing of Disturbed Acceleration

Chapter 5 discussed the method of pretreatment of the output of accelerometer with FIR low-pass filtering. Therefore, low-pass filtering is carried out with FIR filter by selecting appropriate window function.

3. The Inertial Alignment Technology with Digital Filter

After processing the signals of gyroscope and accelerometer with digital filter, we could carry out the initial alignment of inertial system. During the process of alignment, we need to solve the transformational relations between the loading system and launching coordinate system, that is, the initial value of attitude matrix. Assume that the real launching inertial system is $o - xyz$ and the launching coordinate system established by strapdown inertial navigation *Mathematical Platform* is $o - x'y'z'$. After the alignment is completed, commonly there is one small deviation between $o - xyz$ and $o - x'y'z'$, which is called misalignment angle, as shown in Fig. 9.3. The α_0 is the launching azimuth, and β_0 is the latitude of the launch point.

The launching coordinate system rotates in the inertial space along with the Earth. Once the base rocket takes off from Point A, the launching coordinate system at the moment of takeoff is fixed in inertial space, to set up the launching inertial system, as the navigation coordinate system of the flight vehicle during the whole flight process.

It is a remarkable fact that the alignment error is mainly shown by the misalignment angle of the inertial navigation mathematical platform (the specific content refers to the analysis of error of inertial navigation system in Chap. 4). The volume of the misalignment angle is directly correlated with the equivalent deviation of the inertial devices (the volume is commonly at angular component level). During the whole flight process of the OTV, the navigation means that could be used mainly include inertial navigation, satellite navigation, and celestial navigation. The satellite navigation is mainly used for correcting the position and velocity error of inertial navigation, which has limited capability for attitude correction. Before the starlight navigation starts working, the misalignment angle exists all the time. At this moment, the accuracy of initial alignment and the measurement accuracy of gyroscope and accelerometer determine the accuracy of navigation attitude parameters of the flight vehicle. The correction of misalignment angle is mainly carried out with the attitude information output by the starlight navigation after the starlight navigation begins working.

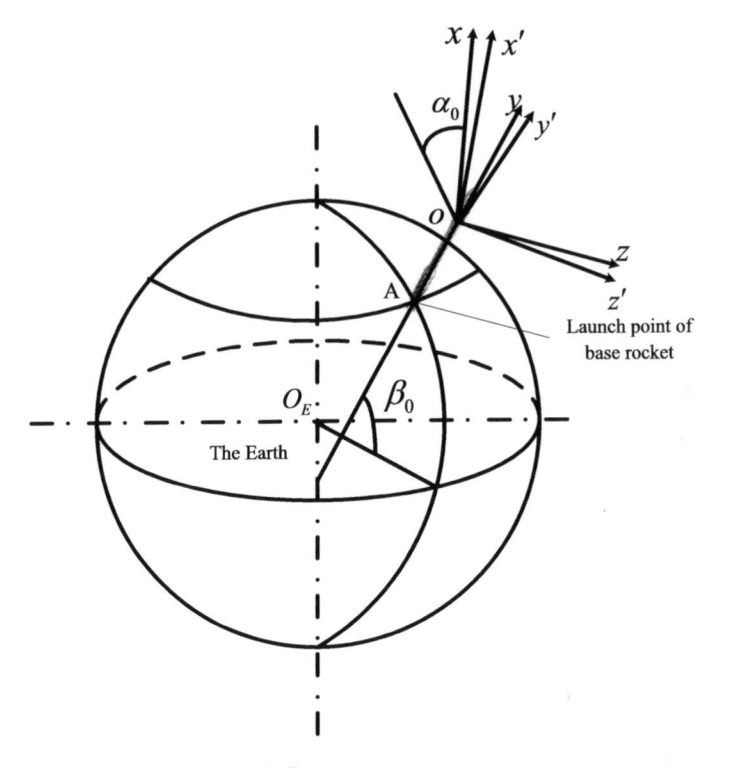

Fig. 9.3 Schematic diagram of initial alignment

9.2.2 Design of INS/GNSS Integrated Navigation

After completing the initial alignment, the base rocket takes off from Point A on the ground by hosting the OTV. After that, the INS/GNSS integrated navigation system of the flight vehicle begins working. To guarantee that the navigation system could work normally when the visible satellites are less than 4, the tightly integrated navigation modes could be used.

During the process from Point A to Point B, since the flight vehicle is hosted on the base rocket for all the time, although the flight vehicle transmits navigation information for all the time, it has not been controlled by the navigation information.

At Point B, the base rocket separates from the flight vehicle. After that, the flight vehicle enters parking orbit and slides to Point C for the first ignition brake. During the process from Point B to C, the flight vehicle calculates the guidance parameters and regulates the attitude properly with the navigation information sent by the INS/GNSS integrated navigation. Such section is mainly making sufficient preparation for the first ignition guidance. After starts guidance from Point C, the information of the INS/GNSS integrated navigation system is similar used for

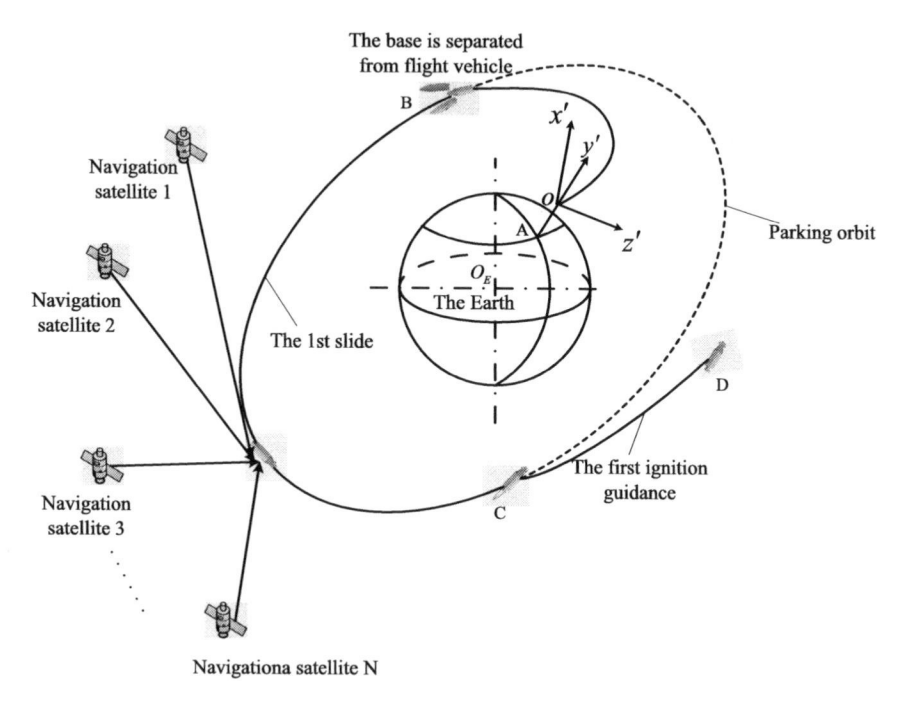

Fig. 9.4 Schematic diagram of INS/GNSS integrated navigation

controlling the flight vehicle until Point D. The first ignition brake is ended. The flight process of such section is shown in Fig. 9.4.

9.2.3   *Reconfiguration of IMU*

As the core navigation system, the INS is working during the whole flight missions. During the process of the base rocket takes off from ground by hosting the OTV to the separation between base rocket and the OTV, that is, the flight process from Point A to Point B, although the OTV itself has not been under control, its INS remains in the working state, calculating the concurrent orbital parameter information in real time. Therefore, the redundant fault tolerance and fault reconfiguration of the inertial system are working during the whole flight missions process from Point A to Point K. The three-orthogonal two-inclined redundant scheme in a single table inertial group described in Chap. 7 could be used for the reconfiguration process of fault detection, isolation, and navigation output signal in three directions (Fig. 9.5).

Fig. 9.5 Schematic diagram
of reconfiguration of IMU

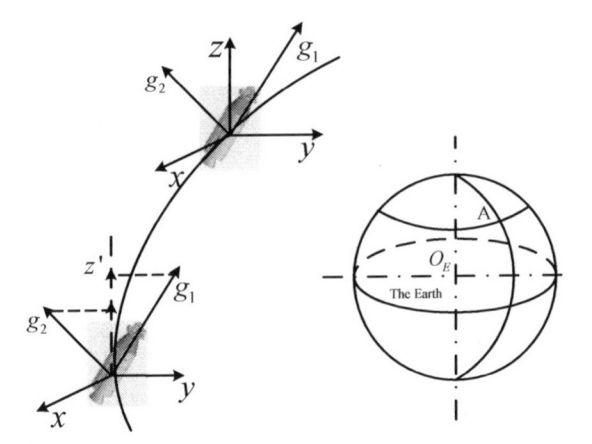

9.2.4 Design of Orbital Prediction

After the first ignition of OTV from Point D to the midcourse correction point E, since the orbital position is lower, the satellite signals received by the flight vehicle are weak and the satellite navigation could not be used for correcting the accumulated error of the inertial navigation tools. The orbital prediction technology

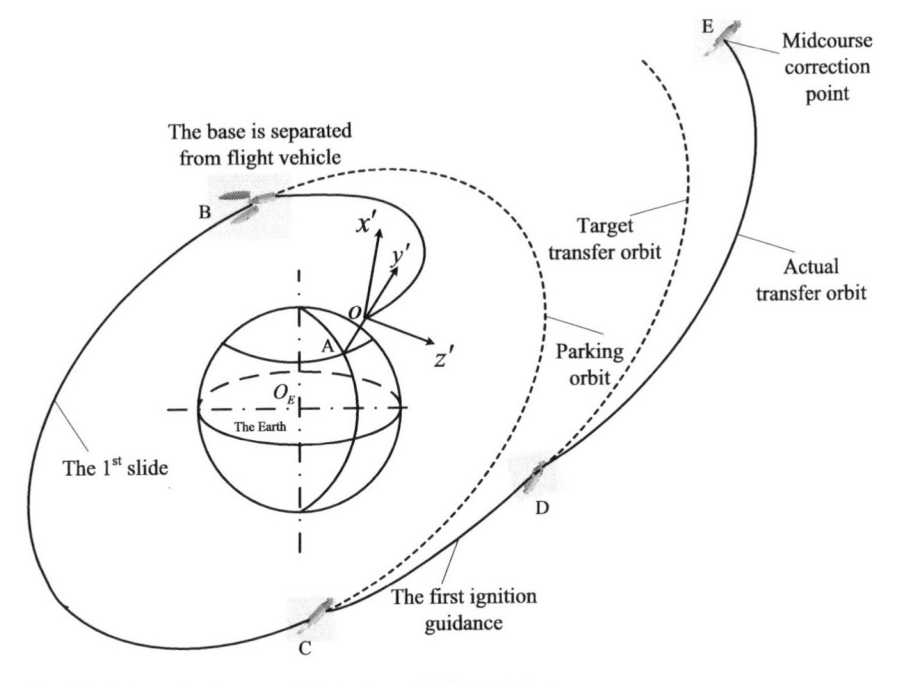

Fig. 9.6 Schematic diagram of designing orbital prediction

shall be used for predicting the orbital parameters from the transfer point D to E, and provides basic orbital parameters for the midcourse correction strategy at Point E. The orbital prediction differential equation takes the centroid motion equation described in Chap. 2, and the initial orbit needed for orbital prediction is obtained from measured data via the process of parameter estimation. The extended Kalman filter method is used for estimating the initial value. Chapter 3 discusses the numerical integration algorithms including Adams method, Cowell method, Adams–Cowell method, and Rung–Kutta method. The multistage Runge–Kutta algorithm could be used for numerical integration (Fig. 9.6).

9.2.5 Design of INS/RCNS Integrated Navigation

After two midcourse corrections, the flight vehicle enters Point H of nominal transfer orbit. At this moment, since the orbital height is higher and unable to receive the signals of navigation satellite, the satellite navigation is out of action. Meanwhile, the orbital height could ensure the flight vehicle away from the atmosphere and observe the star image normally, that is, the starlight navigation system could work normally. During the free sliding process from Point H to Point I, the flight vehicle could correct the inertial navigation by starlight navigation, mainly correct the misalignment angle and the drift error (instrumental error) of the gyroscope after the completion of initial alignment. During the process from Point H to Point I, the flight vehicle calculates the guidance parameters and regulates the attitude appropriately with the navigation information sent by the INS/starlight integrated navigation, which mainly makes full preparation for the second ignition guidance. After begining the guidance at Point I, similarly, the flight vehicle shall be controlled by the information of INS/starlight integrated navigation until Point J, and the second ignition guidance is completed. The flight process of such section is shown in Fig. 9.7.

9.2.6 Design of Midcourse Correction

After completing the first ignition guidance, because of the effects of injection error, navigation error, and thrust deviation of motor, as well as the Earth nonspherical gravitation and lunisolar attraction, there is deviation between the actual transfer orbit of the fight vehicle entered from Point D and the nominal transfer orbit, which needs to be corrected. With the contents described in Chap. 8, first, select two points from actual transfer orbit and nominal transfer orbit, respectively, as the start point and the final target point of correction, and calculate the velocity pulse to be applied for the two midcourse corrections. Then, calculate the switch on and shutdown time of the two corrections according to the specific configuration of

Fig. 9.7 Schematic diagram
of INS/CNS integrated
navigation

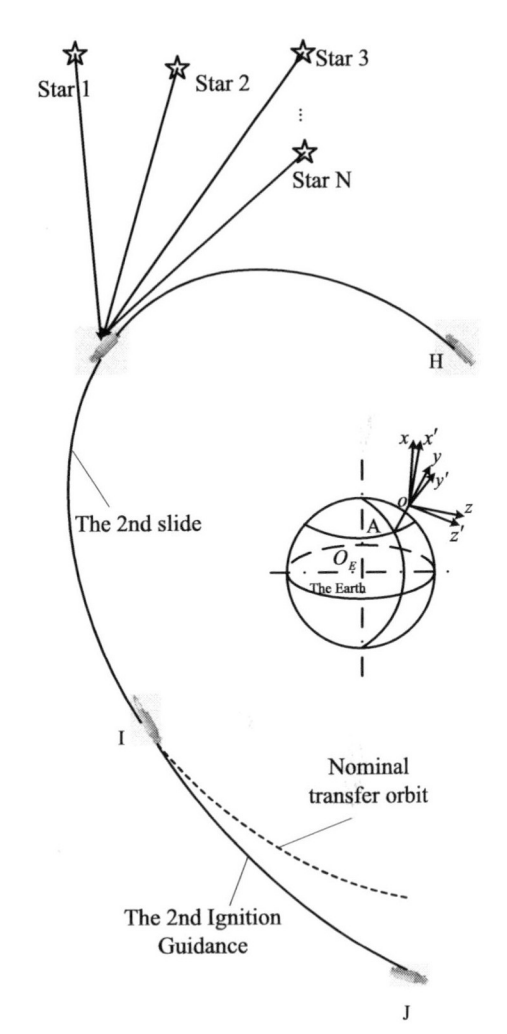

motors. The switch point of the first midcourse correction is the Point E on actual
transfer orbit. After that, it enters the Point F of transition orbit. From then on, the
flight vehicle will slide to Point G of the transition orbit and carry out the second
midcourse correction. After the correction is completed, the flight vehicle enters
Point H of nominal transfer orbit. The flight process of such section is shown in
Fig. 9.8.

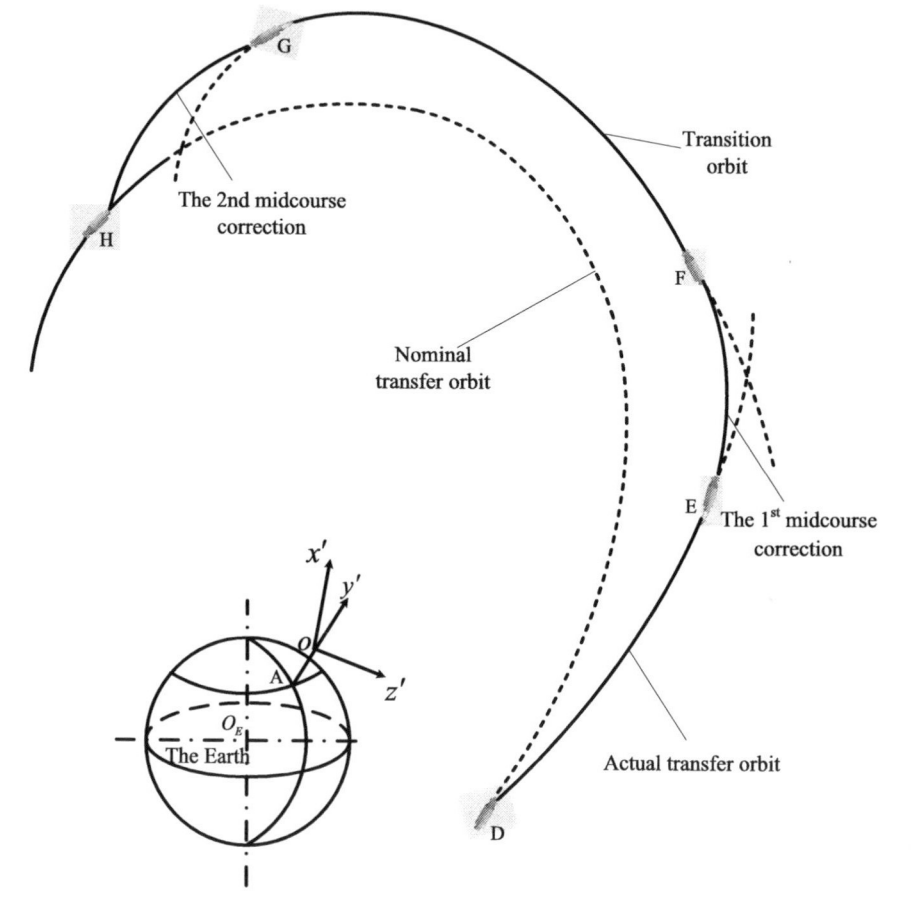

Fig. 9.8 Schematic diagram of midcourse correction

9.2.7 Design of Transfer Orbital Control

The two orbit maneuvers of the flight vehicle are realized by the sustainer motor configured. The specific guidance algorithm adopts the perturbation guidance or iterative guidance described in this chapter. The flight vehicle starts the first ignition guidance at the Point C of the parking orbit. The algorithm of the first ignition guidance adopts the perturbation guidance and the scheme of half-axis shutdown. The flight process of such section is shown in Fig. 9.9.

The flight vehicle begins the second ignition guidance from Point I of the nominal transfer orbit. At this moment, since the orbital height is higher, compared

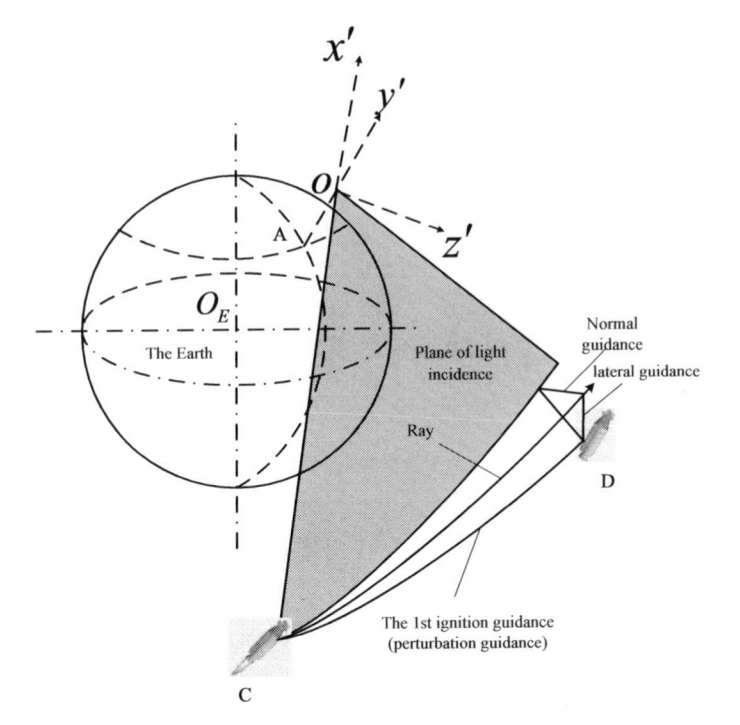

Fig. 9.9 Schematic diagram of the first ignition guidance

to the thrust of the sustainer motor, the proportion of the gravitational force is decreased. Meanwhile, there is no effect from the atmosphere. Thus, the algorithm of the second ignition guidance adopts iterative guidance. The guidance solution is mainly conducted in the orbital coordinate system of the injection point. After obtaining the command of attitude angle in the orbital coordinate system of the injection point, calculate the command of the attitude inside the launching inertial system with a coordinate transformation. Then, track on the command of attitude angle with attitude motor. The flight process of such section is shown in Fig. 9.10. Here, $O_E - x_{ocf}y_{ocf}z_{ocf}$ is the orbital coordinate system of injection point.

After the second ignition guidance is completed, the flight vehicle enters the Point J of the synchronous orbit. When the flight vehicle slides to Point K and releases the payload at Point, the whole flight mission is completed.

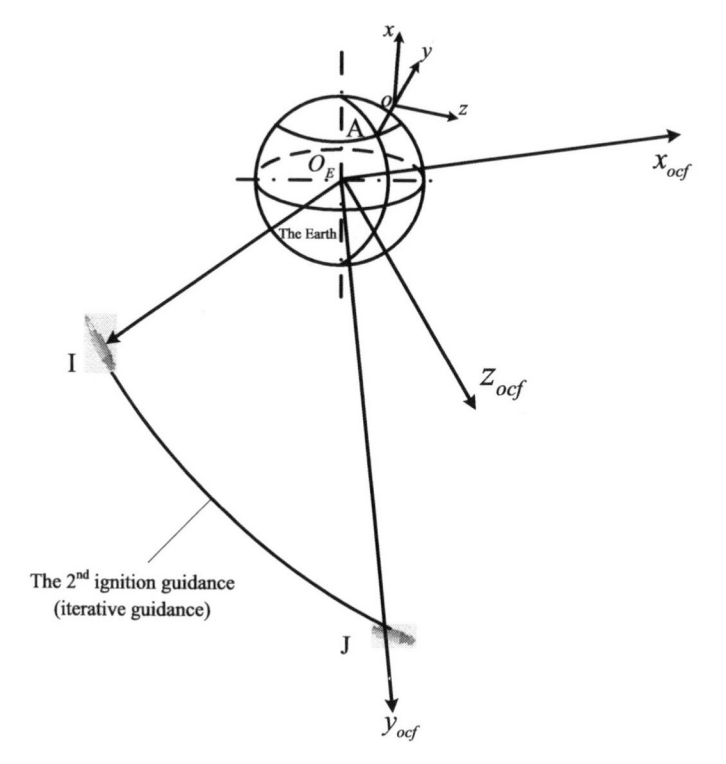

Fig. 9.10 Schematic diagram of the second ignition guidance

Reference Documentation

1. Zhang Wanli. 2011. *Research on Trace Optimization and Guidance Algorithm of Orbital Transfer Vehicle*. Harbin Institute of Technology.
2. Zhong Xiaoli. 2013. *Research on Initial Alignment Method of Rocket-borne Strapdown Inertial Navigation System*. Southeast China University.
3. Liu Bing. 2006. *Research on Orbit Prediction Method of Lunar Spacecraft*. National University of Defense Technology.

Erratum to: Introduction

Erratum to:
Chapter 1 in: X. Li and C. Li, *Navigation and Guidance*
***of Orbital Transfer Vehicle*, Navigation: Science**
and Technology, https://doi.org/10.1007/978-981-10-6334-3_1

In the original version of the book, Fig. 1.1 has been replaced with the new figure in Chapter 1. The erratum chapter and the book have been updated with the change.

The updated online version of this chapter can be found at
https://doi.org/10.1007/978-981-10-6334-3_1

© Springer Nature Singapore Pte Ltd. and National Defense Industry Press, Beijing 2018   E1
X. Li and C. Li, *Navigation and Guidance of Orbital Transfer Vehicle*, Navigation:
Science and Technology, https://doi.org/10.1007/978-981-10-6334-3_10

Printed in Great Britain
by Amazon

80925711R00111